T0146170

A Process Evaluation of Primary Care Behavioral Health Integration in the Military Health System

ANDRADA TOMOAIA-COTISEL, NICOLE K. EBERHART, CHARLES C. ENGEL, PETER MENDEL, GABRIELA ALVARADO, NABEEL SHARIQ QURESHI, SAMUEL D. ALLEN

Prepared for Psychological Health Center of Excellence
Approved for public release; distribution unlimited

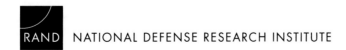

NATIONAL DEFENSE RESEARCH INSTITUTE

For more information on this publication, visit **www.rand.org/t/RRA677-1**.

About RAND

The RAND Corporation is a research organization that develops solutions to public policy challenges to help make communities throughout the world safer and more secure, healthier and more prosperous. RAND is nonprofit, nonpartisan, and committed to the public interest. To learn more about RAND, visit www.rand.org.

Research Integrity

Our mission to help improve policy and decisionmaking through research and analysis is enabled through our core values of quality and objectivity and our unwavering commitment to the highest level of integrity and ethical behavior. To help ensure our research and analysis are rigorous, objective, and nonpartisan, we subject our research publications to a robust and exacting quality-assurance process; avoid both the appearance and reality of financial and other conflicts of interest through staff training, project screening, and a policy of mandatory disclosure; and pursue transparency in our research engagements through our commitment to the open publication of our research findings and recommendations, disclosure of the source of funding of published research, and policies to ensure intellectual independence. For more information, visit www.rand.org/about/principles.

RAND's publications do not necessarily reflect the opinions of its research clients and sponsors.

Published by the RAND Corporation, Santa Monica, Calif.
© 2021 RAND Corporation
RAND® is a registered trademark.

Library of Congress Cataloging-in-Publication Data is available for this publication.
ISBN: 978-1-9774-0713-9

Cover: Drazen - stock.adobe.com.

Limited Print and Electronic Distribution Rights

Preface

Behavioral health (BH) problems are common in the military and can adversely affect force readiness. Research suggests that primary care–behavioral health (PCBH) integration can improve BH outcomes by making high-quality BH care available in more accessible settings. However, sustaining high-quality implementation of PCBH is challenging. The authors conducted a process evaluation of the PCBH program in the military health system to understand why the program is working as it is and provide recommendations for quality improvement. They conducted semistructured interviews, rigorously coded the qualitative data to identify causal links, and created and validated causal loop diagrams that provide a visualization of how the system is working.

The research reported here was completed in December 2020 and underwent security review with the sponsor before public release.

This research was sponsored by the Psychological Health Center of Excellence and conducted within the Forces and Resources Policy (FRP) Center of the RAND National Security Research Division, which operates the National Defense Research Institute, a federally funded research and development center sponsored by the Office of the Secretary of Defense, the Joint Staff, the Unified Combatant Commands, the Navy, the Marine Corps, the defense agencies, and the defense intelligence enterprise.

For more information on the RAND FRP Center, see www.rand.org/nsrd/frp or contact the director (contact information is provided on the webpage).

Contents

Figures and Table

Figures

Table

Summary

Behavioral health (BH) problems are common in the military and can adversely affect force readiness. Research suggests that primary care–behavioral health (PCBH) integration can improve BH outcomes by making high-quality BH care available in more accessible settings. However, sustaining high-quality implementation of PCBH is challenging. We conducted a process evaluation of the PCBH program in the military health system to understand why the program is working as it is. We conducted semistructured interviews, rigorously coded the qualitative data to identify causal links, and created and validated causal loop diagrams that provide a visualization of how the system is working.

We provide findings in four key areas: staffing and capabilities, valued tasks, program stewardship, and fostering program awareness and support. Adequate *staffing*—meaning the right level and with the right capabilities—is crucial to the success of PCBH. This adequate staffing can be achieved by retaining existing staff and hiring when needed. Retention, in turn, is driven by staff and supervisor satisfaction, reflected in adherence to the model (which local leaders interpret as productivity and number of visits per patient, among other factors). When leadership works actively to improve staff satisfaction and adherence to the model, it is supporting PCBH staff retention. When staff are hired, those with more PCBH-relevant capabilities are more likely to succeed in the role, thus improving retention. While some sites regarded General Schedule (GS) staffing as the potential solution to staffing issues because of flexibility in managing and incentivizing staff, it also can create administrative burdens.

Patient care consists of providing direct patient care, bridging care with other providers, providing consultations to other staff members, and group classes. However, there are other *valued tasks* in addition to patient care, such as conducting screenings, fostering awareness of the PCBH program, and charting or other documentation. All of these together make up the PCBH staff workload, and when the workload becomes too high, staff responds by either limiting associated valued tasks or encouraging fewer referrals. If these compensation mechanisms do not work, staff members get burned out, which places a higher burden on staff that work closely with them, and if they leave the position, the workload of those remaining will be further increased.

Local leadership acts as *stewards* of the program by maintaining staffing and capability levels. This is accomplished by hiring new staff when needed, working to improve scope of work and benefits packages, being a good and supportive manager, and working with staff to understand the model of care. These activities are conducted depending on leadership perceptions of adherence to the model and retention. The success of the PCBH program also relies on having *supportive stakeholders*. Primary care managers (PCMs) buy into the program when they are fully aware of it and can see that it works. Teamwork, understanding the model, and routine day-to-day promotion bolster PCM support, while behavioral health consultant (BHC) turnover makes it more challenging to maintain support.

We identified recommendations to improve program implementation, and we present them according to the four key results areas.

PCBH Staffing and Capabilities

- **Improve job descriptions**. This will ensure that applicants have a comprehensive understanding of the positions and can better self-assess whether they are a good match for the job. We suggest ensuring that job descriptions convey the high volume of clinical work (i.e., large number of brief appointments) and clearly lay out nonclinical duties. We further suggest putting pressure on local installation contracting offices to, in turn, pressure contracting organizations to accurately convey what the positions entail.
- **Improve contracting process and/or transition key PCBH staff positions to GS.** It may be possible to work with installation contracting offices to put pressure on contractors to reduce turnover and to incorporate management tools into contracts. If it is not possible to improve the contracting process, we recommend transitioning key PCBH positions to GS.
- **Prioritize rapid rehiring.** This will minimize gaps in service as well as ensure that the staff role continues to be valued.

Valued Tasks

- **Identify, count, and reinforce valued tasks.** We recommend identifying all valued tasks and giving them increased visibility, protecting and dedicating time for them, and targeting them in routine, *ongoing* training.
- **Continue to work toward awareness of tasks and roles—beyond BHC.** We recommend increasing efforts to promote understanding of the behavioral health care facilitator (BHCF) role and local (clinic and installation) leadership roles.

PCBH Stewardship

- **Increase support for local leadership.** We recommend increasing orientation and ongoing communication with local leaders regarding their role and assisting local leadership in helping BHCs and BHCFs in fostering awareness of the PCBH program.
- **Implement routine measurement and monitoring of *comprehensive* metrics.** We recommend that central program leadership and local installation leadership routinely use a comprehensive set of implementation metrics and performance objectives in assessing how things are going and providing sites with more training on how to use these metrics.

We further suggest setting *trip wires* that flag need for action (e.g., for BHC workload, decreased PCM referrals).

- **Cultivate local champions.** We recommend that the PCBH managers increase their efforts to identify and cultivate installation-level champions.
- **Increase central support for local PCBH staff.** We recommend efforts to continuously build BHC skills so that staff members are comfortable treating the full range of conditions—and PCMs are comfortable referring for a full breadth of conditions—as well as regular and ongoing support for BHCs and BHCFs and orientation for PCMs.

Fostering PCBH Awareness and Support

- **Provide more central assistance in fostering awareness of the PCBH program.** We recommend increasing support for local leadership in routinely promoting close teamwork and awareness of PCBH. We further recommend that central program leaders do more to promote program awareness, such as regularly updating and disseminating centrally developed promotional materials for both BHC and BHCF services.

Acknowledgments

We would like to acknowledge the contributions of the program officer (Justin Curry) and PCBH-related Defense Health Agency personnel in providing periodic feedback throughout this process evaluation. We would also like to thank the installation-level personnel who gave their time to participate in interviews discussing their experiences with the PCBH program. This evaluation and report were improved by the contributions of our quality assurance reviewers, Lisa Meredith, William L. Miller, and Craig Bond.

Abbreviations

BH	behavioral health
BHC	behavioral health consultant
BHCF	behavioral health care facilitator
BHI	behavioral health integration
BHIP	Behavioral Health Integration Program
BHM	Behavioral Health Monitor
BHOP	Behavioral Health Optimization Program
CBT	cognitive behavioral therapy
CLD	causal loop diagram
COVID-19	coronavirus disease 2019
DCoE	Defense Center of Excellence
DHA	Defense Health Agency
DoD	Department of Defense
GS	General Schedule
MH	mental health
MHS	Military Health System
MTF	military treatment facility
OIC	officer in charge
PCBH	primary care behavioral health
PCM	primary care manager
PCMH	patient-centered medical home
PTSD	posttraumatic stress disorder

RESPECT-Mil   Re-Engineering Systems of Primary Care Treatment of PTSD and
                     Depression in the Military
STEPS-UP   Stepped Enhancement of PTSD Services Using Primary Care
VA   U.S. Department of Veterans Affairs

CHAPTER ONE

Introduction

Background

Access to high-quality primary care management of behavioral health (BH) conditions is a high priority for the U.S. Military Health System (MHS). Military personnel face operational and traumatic stressors that can place them at elevated risk for common mental health problems, such as depression, anxiety, and posttraumatic stress disorder (PTSD) (Stahlman and Oetting, 2018; Kessler et al., 2014; Rosellini et al., 2015), as well as a wide range of other BH issues, such as chronic pain (Toblin et al., 2014), alcohol and tobacco misuse (e.g., Meadows et al., 2018), poor sleep hygiene (Troxel et al., 2015), and overweight status (e.g., Rush, Leard-Mann, and Crum-Cianflone, 2016). These BH issues are prevalent and frequently overlap in primary care patients seen in the military, Department of Veterans Affairs (VA), and nonfederal health care settings (Gillock et al., 2005; Gureje et al., 1998; Hoge et al., 2007; Kroenke et al., 2007; Lazar, 2014; Liebschutz et al., 2007; Toblin et al., 2014).

BH conditions are often disabling; contribute to military attrition, absenteeism, misconduct, and sick call visits; increase the use of costly medical resources; and represent a threat to military readiness (Eibner et al., 2008; Hoge, Lesikar, and Guevara, 2002; Hoge et al., 2007). In part due to military culture—with its emphasis on leadership, team over individual, and performance under pressure—the stigma associated with BH issues and related suffering can be significant (Acosta et al., 2014; Sharp et al., 2015). This may be further exacerbated for service members who are concerned about limits to privacy and confidentiality of BH treatment in the MHS, where roughly one-third of all service members agree with the statement that seeking BH treatment will damage a service member's military career (Meadows, Miller, and Robson, 2015; Meadows et al., 2021).

These considerations point to the opportunity for primary care to serve as an essential component of the military BH safety net. Less than half of affected serving military personnel receive military mental health services, and often services are not timely or adequate (Colpe et al., 2015; Hoge et al., 2014; Meadows et al., 2018; Tanielian and Jaycox, 2008). While the proportion of service members seeking BH services in a military specialty clinic has varied with the tempo of operations between 8 percent and 22 percent (Hoge, Lesikar, and Guevara, 2002; Hoge, Auchterlonie, and Milliken, 2006), nearly every service member receives some general health care at a military treatment facility (MTF) each year. These services include Pre- and Post-Deployment Health Assessments, an annual Periodic Health Assessment, routine wellness care, obstetrical care, preventive vaccine care, care for minor training injuries, and care for more serious health problems.

The U.S. military has been quick to recognize the potential for BH integration (BHI) as a way of increasing the reach of BH care to those with unmet treatment needs (Engel, Kroenke, and Katon, 1994; Engel, 1994; Harris and LeFavour, 2005; Runyan et al., 2003), and early pockets of expertise rapidly gave way to several ambitious implementation efforts. The first system-wide BHI program implementation occurred in the Air Force, which in 2000 launched the Behavioral Health Optimization Program (BHOP) (Hunter et al., 2014). In the BHOP model, a BH specialist—most often a clinical psychologist, less frequently a social worker—is stationed in the primary care clinic and serves as an active member of the primary care treatment team. This onsite BH specialist—or BH consultant (BHC)—offers clinical consultation and support to primary care providers and their patients. Primary care providers can easily consult BHCs in real time, and BHCs can focus on a broad swath of BH issues, including depression and anxiety, smoking cessation, weight control, and adherence to medical treatment. Primary care providers like the easy access to specialist support for mental health crises, suicide risk assessment, and other problems (Hunter et al., 2014). After some positive experiences deploying psychologists on aircraft carriers, the Navy commissioned a study of BHI that recommended the initiation of a pilot program (Harris and Tela, 2002). In 2003, the Navy launched the Behavioral Health Integration Program (BHIP) in close consultation with the Air Force, adopting a similar primary care behavioral health (PCBH) approach using a modified version of the BHOP program manual. This pilot was discontinued in 2005 because of the rising tempo of operations in Iraq and Afghanistan and the demand for more BH specialists in direct support of those fighting in these conflicts (Hunter et al., 2014).

In 2004, the Army began to pilot RESPECT-Mil (Re-Engineering Systems of Primary Care Treatment in the Military) at Fort Bragg, North Carolina (Engel et al., 2008). The RESPECT-Mil approach to BHI differed significantly from the PCBH approach used by the Air Force and Navy. RESPECT-Mil was based on a *collaborative care* model, an integration that relies on nonspecialist care managers located in primary care settings to engage patients in evidence-based treatment using telephonic and other remote strategies and completing validated measures of symptom severity to track treatment response and enable timely adjustment of treatment. The BH specialist in collaborative care models—most often a psychiatrist, sometimes a psychiatric nurse practitioner—operates off-site, covers a number of clinics, is purely consultative, and seldom provides direct care. Instead, the BH specialist meets individually with each care manager about once a week, reviews panel-based information from electronic health record registries that have been further populated with care manager curated process (e.g., adherence, side effects, time since last contact) and outcome data (e.g., depression, anxiety, pain), and identifies patients who are not responding to treatment or show evidence of other unmet BH needs. Recommendations are discussed with the care manager and relayed to the primary care treatment team. Collaborative care models have been used almost exclusively in the large body of randomized controlled trials investigating BHI to date and emphasize measurement; in that sense, these are highly credible approaches to BHI. However, these collaborative care trials and programs tend to focus in on a narrower subset of BH conditions and clinical outcomes than the more expansive PCBH approach. These models can be less attractive to primary care providers if they do not offer them on-site BH specialist support.

RESPECT-Mil's *multiplier effect*, allowing one BH specialist to cover many clinics, was a selling point as the operational tempo increased. The program was based on RESPECT-Depression, an experimental collaborative care approach designed and tested by MacArthur Foundation–funded researchers to improve outcomes for primary care patients with major depression in civilian settings (Dietrich et al., 2014; Oxman et al., 2002). RESPECT-Mil added PTSD and primary care screening for both conditions at every primary care visit and for suicidal ideation when a screen was positive. In 2007, an Army Surgeon General directive was issued to implement RESPECT-Mil across 42 primary care clinics at 15 installations with deployment platforms, and, in 2010, the program was expanded to include 93 clinics across 40 worldwide installations. Approximately 3.2 million primary care visits were screened for PTSD and depression in RESPECT-Mil: 13 percent screened positive for PTSD or depression, 0.7 percent had suicidal ideation, about 2 percent were referred to specialty BH care, and another 2 percent received primary care case management (Hunter et al., 2014; Wong, Jaycox, and Ayer, 2015). Perceptions of the program among primary care and BH providers and Army Medical Department leaders were generally, though not universally, positive (Wong, Jaycox, and Ayer, 2015).

From 2009 to 2015, RESPECT-Mil program leaders and collaborators at RTI International, RAND Corporation, Uniformed Services University, University of Washington, and Boston University completed a six-installation (18–primary care clinic) randomized trial of a second-generation collaborative care intervention called STEPS-UP (Stepped Enhancement of PTSD Services Using Primary Care), developed from RESPECT-Mil lessons learned. STEPS-UP added stepped remote psychosocial interventions—such as remote case management, interapy, and telephonic cognitive behavioral therapy (CBT)—and face-to-face therapy in primary care (see Engel et al., 2014, for a detailed description of the research and intervention design). After 12 months, STEPS-UP patients showed measurable and statistically significant improvements over those in RESPECT-Mil with regard to both PTSD and depression symptom severity outcomes (Engel et al., 2016).

In 2012, a major reconfiguration of primary care service delivery was initiated in accordance with emerging notions of the patient-centered medical home (PCMH). This created what has been described as a "blended" BHI model, known as *PCBH*. PCBH combines the best elements and lessons learned from the BHOP, BHIP, and RESPECT-Mil models with its reliance on a co-located BH specialist in each clinic to increase primary care provider and patient access to BH care, and its use of a co-located care manager and off-site psychiatric input.

In the years since then, some variation in program implementation has developed. Recently, the MHS is again facing reorganization, this time as a single system under the Defense Health Agency (DHA)—instead of the long tradition of somewhat separate Army, Navy, and Air Force health systems. RAND researchers have been asked to assess and review the implementation of the PCBH program and to provide recommendations with regard to program implementation moving forward.

Our Charge

The RAND team conducted a process evaluation of the PCBH program in the MHS. The goal of the evaluation was to understand the facilitators and challenges of program implementation. We sought to go beyond describing the program to providing an understanding of why the program is functioning as it is, enabling us to provide actionable recommendations for program implementation and quality improvement. The ultimate goal was to facilitate delivery of BH care services in primary care, so that patients receive more effective care.

Organization of This Report

Chapter Two presents our research methods, Chapter Three presents results, and Chapter Four presents conclusions and recommendations.

Methods

Introduction to Causal Loop Diagrams

This evaluation used causal loop diagrams (CLDs) in its analysis of how the PCBH program was functioning. CLDs are a visual representation or "mental map" of how different elements in a system are related to one another. This systematic qualitative approach, based in System Dynamics (Sterman, 2000), is designed to identify and map causal links among components within complex programs (e.g., Fredericks, Deegan, and Carman, 2008). In other words, CLDs draw out how aspects of program implementation are connected to one another, allowing us to see the causes and consequences of each aspect. CLDs visually represent the causal feedback loops we find in these connections, allowing us to make sense of the *why* behind complex situations. This improved understanding helps minimize unintended consequences in program management.

Past Use of CLDs in the Military

CLDs have been used to help solve complex problems in the military. For example, in 1970, Ingalls Shipbuilding won a contract to build destroyers for the U.S. Navy (Sterman, 2000). Six years later, the project experienced millions of dollars in cost overruns. CLDs were used as part of a set of systems tools to identify the causes of delays and cost overruns.

One lesson learned was the importance of *fixes that fail*. Small ship-design changes from the Navy led to ripple effects that drastically disrupted the production system at Ingalls. As the project fell behind schedule, employees were pressured to work overtime to catch up. Apparent productivity gains brought with them an unanticipated side effect: employee fatigue, leading to more mistakes. Simply put—haste made waste.

Conceiving of this situation as a set of causal feedback loops was a key step in identifying leverage points for preventing similar situations. It provided a new way of thinking—the indirect effects of design changes were no longer thought of as producing a small additional cost, but rather as part of an explicit feedback structure causing a cost many times larger than the direct effects. The CLD approach is still used inside and outside government to clarify mechanisms behind system challenges and leverage points for intervention in complex organizational situations.

Overview of How CLDs Were Used in the Current Evaluation

By interviewing across role type within the PCBH program, at different sites, and within different military branches, we were able to build a shared mental model of PCBH implementation that facilitates understanding of how different elements interact with each other and what direct consequences emerge from increasing or decreasing a particular element within the system. This evaluation applied a rigorous mixed methods (Fetters, Curry, and Creswell, 2013; Ivankova, Creswell, and Stick, 2006) approach to developing CLDs (Tomoaia-Cotisel, 2018). It started with gathering stories of what happened and why. Analysis of interview data was focused on mapping out the system behind program implementation: What makes the program work? What makes it fail? What makes it more difficult? To do this, we rigorously coded interview transcripts to find causal links. We brought together diverse perspectives by combining causal links from coded interviews in a diagram, in tandem with a systematic validation process. The final product was a comprehensive CLD visually representing the causal links identified in participants' stories, the collective mental model of program staff.

Interview Participants

Sampling was designed to capture diverse perspectives, to get a comprehensive understanding of the facilitators and challenges involved in PCBH implementation. We sampled nine installations (three Air Force, three Army, and three Navy installations) of different sizes and with diverse PCBH experiences. Installations were selected with input from program managers in each of the three military services, drawing on their knowledge of installations' implementation experiences and context. This selection was also informed by analysis of cross-sectional data about PCBH at all installations. Cross-sectional analysis included service-specific cluster analysis to group sites according to the manner in which they adhere to program guidelines and protocols (e.g., percentage for which BHCs provided feedback to the referring primary care provider), as well as consideration for installation context (e.g., population breakdown between active duty, family of active duty, and retired).[1] Analysis results are from the CLD analysis (see section below); quantitative data were not used beyond informing site selection, which was done collaboratively with PCBH program managers in light of qualitative information they provided on the different sites. We report recommendations derived from experiences shared in qualitative interviews and CLD-based policy analysis.

We interviewed 61 personnel at these installations (equating to 58 interviews, because three interviews had two participants in the interview). The goal for selecting participants was to obtain diverse perspectives on the PCBH program at each installation. Individual partici-

---

[1] We grouped sites into clusters according to how they practice, specifically the percentage of visits in which the BHC communicated with the primary care manager (PCM; PCM Box is checked), percentage of visits in which the Behavioral Health Monitor (BHM-20) was used, and percentage of visits in which any symptom-specific checklist was used. We also examined BHC visit characteristics such as number of visits per patient, range of conditions treated by a BHC, visit code used most, average number of services per visit, and number of visits per day. We examined site-level characteristics, including the size of the BHC population and total population, as well as percentage of BHC patients and all patients who are active duty, retired, and family of active duty. Our analysis found seven distinct ways BHCs practiced. These seven groups did not correlate to BHCs' visit, patient, or site characteristics. Thus, all of these criteria were useful in preparing recommendations for site selection, which was done in consultation with PCBH program managers. Behavioral health outcomes data were not used for selection.

pants were identified by installation-level staff. Table 2.1 summarizes PCBH program roles and interview participants.

Protocol Development and Data Collection

The RAND team developed the PCBH Logic Model collaboratively, with input from the program managers in charge of PCBH implementation, the PCBH program developers, and Defense Center of Excellence (DCoE) staff members. This Logic Model was used to inform the development of evaluation questions and, consequently, data collection instruments (see Appendix A).

The study team developed four sets of interview guides: one for BHCs, one for BHCFs, one for PCMs, and one for leadership personnel at the installation. Each interview guide focused on the participant's role in and experiences with the PCBH program—stories of what happened and why. Participants answered open-ended questions about their PCBH implementation experiences. Interviewers then probed more deeply to ask for causes and implications. Copies of the interview guides are available from the authors upon request.

Interviews were semistructured, given that question wording and probes were tailored to the context and expertise of the stakeholders. Interviews lasted approximately 45 minutes. Most interviews were conducted via telephone, and interviews were audio-recorded (with participant permission) and transcribed for analysis, except in cases where the participant did not give this permission; in such cases, detailed manual notes were taken and used in the analysis. Interviews for one Navy installation were conducted during an in-person site visit, but coronavirus disease 2019 (COVID-19) travel restrictions precluded planned in-person data collection at Army and Air Force sites. In addition, some potential participants declined to be interviewed because they were occupied addressing COVID-19–related needs at their installations.

Note that our approach focusing on interviews was limited, to the extent that interviews reflect perceptions rather than actual behavior. We were able to collect observational data from one site, but COVID-19 precluded additional site visits. We also reviewed program documents

Table 2.1
Interview Participants

Role	Description	N
BHCs	Psychologists and social workers who provide consultation, assessment, and brief intervention for a wide range of BH conditions, as well as chronic health problems and problematic health behaviors	18
Behavioral health care facilitators (BHCFs)	Care managers (typically registered nurses) who support treatment of individuals with depression, anxiety, or PTSD by encouraging treatment adherence and monitoring treatment response	10
PCMs	Primary care providers who work together with BHCs, BHCFs, and other staff to provide comprehensive treatment for patients	16
Local leaders	Individuals who play an administrative role in the PCBH program, such as the Officer in Charge (OIC) of a clinic or the PCBH champion for an installation	14
	Total	**61**

NOTE: Some participants were local installation-level leaders as well as service providers (e.g., PCMs). In these cases, they were counted only once, and they were counted as "local leaders."

to understand how interviews fit with program materials, although the data analysis was based solely on interview data, as described in the following section.

Data Analysis

Data analysis focused on mapping out the system behind PCBH program implementation.

Interview transcripts were rigorously coded to identify the variables and causal links inside the stories that participants shared. The evaluation team went through iterative rounds of coding that began with identifying causal language in the text data. We developed a coding scheme using interviews from one installation and refined it as needed as new concepts arose in coding data from additional installations. This coding scheme did more than just identify elements: Excerpts of causal language were converted into simple CLD-type word and arrow diagrams to identify the variable being discussed *and* to signify the direction in which causality flows. An example of this type of coding is presented in Appendix B. A quality assurance process was followed throughout the coding process. Each interview transcript was coded by one of three coders. Initial coder training consisted of independently coding transcripts at one installation, then reviewing and discussing coding performed. This involved an interrater reliability assessment and periodic review of coding performed.

We brought together diverse perspectives by combining causal links from coded interviews into a diagram. The result of this merging was a comprehensive CLD visually representing the causal links identified in participants' stories.

Saturation tests were implemented during data analysis: first using interviews from one installation from each service (n = 22 interviews) and second using the remaining interviews (n = 36 interviews). Saturation was reached both times. The first test informed the decision to conclude initial conceptualization of a tentative model. This allowed us to move from using a coding process designed to rigorously document each variable and link to a similar process that explicitly searches for disconfirming evidence in subsequent interviews. The second test informed the decision to confidently move from model development to model use (i.e., from conducting interviews and identifying and linking variables in a CLD to interpreting the CLD and identifying policy recommendations).

We walked through this CLD with experts in BHI in military primary care. They included members of the broader research team, RAND's internal quality assurance reviewers, and BH leaders in each of the three military services. The purpose of these discussions was to check that it made sense to them and make clarifications as needed. The resulting CLD is presented in Figures 3.25 through 3.27 in Chapter Three. We also generated Shared Understanding Diagrams to document the extent to which each link in the CLD was mentioned across all interview participants of a specific group. These results are presented by service (Army, Navy, Air Force) and by the participant's primary role for the interviews (BHC, BHCF, PCM, local leader) in Appendix C.

Orientation to CLDs

Because we use CLDs to describe the findings, we provide a brief orientation to them here. This description accompanies Figure 2.1:

Figure 2.1
A CLD Example

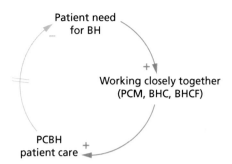

- **Words** on the diagram indicate variables representing important facts and concepts (for example, *resources, perceptions, decisions, goals*)
- **Arrows** indicate *cause-effect* links. This is the way a change in one variable leads another variable to change, so, for example, a + indicates same-direction change, and a – indicates opposite-direction change. Positive links are shown as blue arrows and negative links as pink arrows.
- **Double hash marks** indicate *delays*, a type of causal link in which it takes more time for the effect to be perceived. Delays are important because they are the reason why we can't easily see the effects of our actions, which is one reason why CLDs can be helpful.
- **Loops** indicate a causal chain that feeds back on itself over time, in which a change is either reinforced or counteracted over time. Any one loop can tell what happens when a variable in that loop increases, and what happens when a variable in that loop decreases over time—in so doing, it is able to capture multiple stories about the same system.

CHAPTER THREE

Results

We begin by presenting the balancing loop at the core of the PCBH program. Next, we present how facilitators and barriers affect this central loop to destabilize and/or support PCBH. These are organized in four topics: *staffing and capabilities, valued tasks, PCBH stewardship,* and *fostering PCBH awareness and support.* Because these topics are interdependent, the section for each topic includes some information about other topics. After laying out how PCBH works in these four topics, we describe the important role that PCMs play. We conclude this section by giving an overview of the overarching CLD that brings all of these topics together.

The Core of the PCBH Program Is Staff Working Together to Meet Patient Behavioral Health Needs

Participants reported that, at its core, PCBH addresses patient needs. Primary care patients present with BH needs. When needs begin to increase, BHCs and BHCFs respond by working closely with each other and with PCMs (specific tasks are identified in the "valued tasks" section). As they work closely together, they provide more patient care. Over time (see delay mark on Figure 3.1), providing more PCBH patient care works to counter the increase in patients' BH needs. Alternatively, when team members believe that patients' BH needs are decreasing, they work less closely together, they provide less care, and, over time, PCBH contributes less to meeting patients' needs.

This loop shows the core of the program. The PCBH program is essentially a balancing loop that seeks to maintain patient behavioral health needs under control.

Figure 3.1
PCBH Meets Patients' Behavioral Health Needs

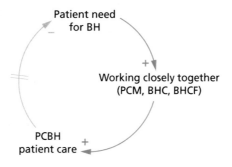

PCBH Staffing and Capabilities

Adequate PCBH Staffing Is Crucial to PCBH Success

Figure 3.2 extends the core loop in Figure 3.1 (now shown with bolded arrows to indicate that these are all links that we have covered in a previous figure). Adequate PCBH staffing is crucial to PCBH success because it affects the day-to-day PCBH work. By *adequate*, we are referring both to the right level of staffing and to the right capabilities of staff to ensure PCBH success. An adequate level of staff should be able to perform all the tasks that are necessary for PCBH success—this may or may not match the staffing formula in program doctrine because not all tasks that participants described as being crucial to success are counted at present in that doctrine (see "valued tasks" section).

Figure 3.2
PCBH Staffing Influences Workload, Teamwork, and Patient Care

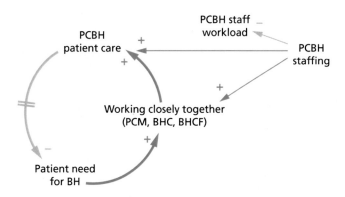

NOTE: Thick arrows are links already present in prior figures.

Adequate PCBH staffing is crucial because having many staff members at a site is a necessary precondition to those staff working closely together (both BHCs with BHCFs and PCBH staff with PCMs), thereby providing more patient care. Having more staff also reduces the workload on PCBH staff so that they have more time for valued activities. This situation is summarized by one PCM as follows:

> I need more people. [. . .] I think part of what goes bad is they say, 'OK now you're going to do this' and then there's nobody to do it.

Adequate PCBH staffing is obtained through retention of existing staff and hiring of new staff when needed; see Figure 3.3. Hiring of PCBH staff occurs because local leadership is engaged in stewardship over the PCBH program at the installation. This hiring process takes time (more on that in the "PCBH stewardship" section).

It is important to note that participants whom we interviewed at some of the installations indicated that, while they might have had a BHCF previously, their sites did not have a BHCF at the time and did not plan to hire one in the future (see "Fostering PCBH awareness and support" section), even though the program requires BHCFs for installations of that size.

Figure 3.3
Retention Quickly Changes Staffing, and Hiring Takes Time

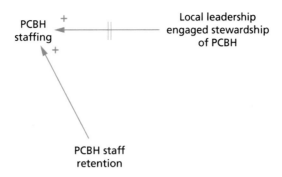

PCBH Staff Retention Is Driven by Staff and Supervisor Satisfaction

PCBH staff are retained when they choose to stay and when their supervisors wish them to stay (Figure 3.4). PCBH staff choose to stay when they are satisfied with the day-to-day work. PCBH staff also choose to stay when their jobs are as they expected—both the day-to-day tasks and the benefits package. For example, several PCBH staff members across installations highlighted that having stable benefit packages with enough leave and flexibility for overtime made them more likely to remain in their positions. This aspect was especially concerning for PCBH staff hired using contractor organizations (i.e., non–General Schedule (GS); more on this in the "Using contracting organizations" section).

Figure 3.4
Factors Informing PCBH Staff Retention

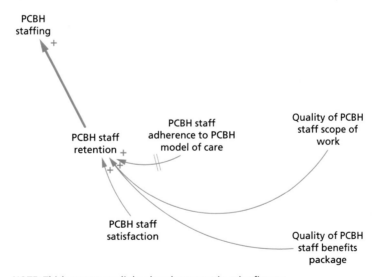

NOTE: Thick arrows are links already present in prior figures.

Supervisors of PCBH staff wish to retain them when they adhere to the model. There are two important caveats here. First, staff may choose to leave before they are formally fired, but the idea is the same—that their lack of adherence to the model is what makes them leave. Second, supervisors are not always PCBH stewards (see next section). Sometimes, the assigned supervisors may provide the clinical oversight necessary but not engage in assessing and addressing adherence to the PCBH model. Indeed, sometimes, supervisors cause PCBH staff to diverge from the model.

An installation-level PCBH lead recounted:

> I had a provider that was exceeding that [maximum number of visits per patient in the model], going up to 14 to 23 visits [per patient]. . . . [we communicated] that back to the [central leadership], that the limits [had] been exceeded and . . . that was communicated back to the contractor. The employee was warned and . . . before he got fired, he quit.

Local Leadership at the Installation Support PCBH Staff Retention When Leaders Work to Improve PCBH Staff Adherence and Satisfaction

To expand on this experience just described, the engaged PCBH lead should not fire the non-adherent PCBH staff member. The PCBH lead ideally notices the lack of adherence and works to help the PCBH staff member to better understand what their role entails. If the PCBH staff member adapts his work to better follow the model, then the PCBH lead is able to reduce further engagement (Figure 3.5).

Figure 3.5
Local Leaders Work to Improve Understanding of the PCBH Model and PCBH Staff Satisfaction

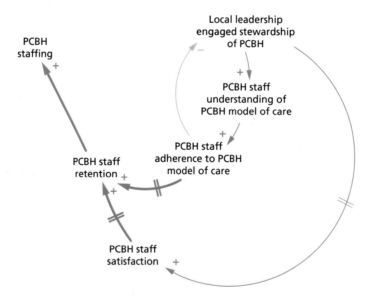

NOTE: Thick arrows are links already present in prior figures.

A BHC described an experience in which PCBH staff were retained through the mechanism. In this case, the OIC at the clinic engaged not only with the BHC but also with the PCMs at the clinic to improve adherence to the PCBH model of care.

When [the OIC] wanted to change my schedule to say ten scheduled patients, I probably would have lost my mind; but he explained it to me and why we're trying to do [it]. . . . So we're going to schedule me for ten a day, [which] is going to be hectic, but that's to hold the PCMs' feet to the fire, to make sure they're sending the referrals because if I got ten available slots a day, and they're not filled up because docs are not sending me people, then that way he can address that with them. . . . He's the model chief.

This experience also shows one way that local leadership can improve satisfaction: by listening to PCBH staff concerns and working to address problems (in this case, the low level of referrals from PCMs and the BHC's fears about burnout). Staff also reported that local leaders can improve satisfaction with quality improvement projects.

These are just a few of the ways local leadership engages in stewardship of PCBH—others are covered in the PCBH stewardship section that follows.

Past Related Experience and Patient Need Can Also Cause Staff to Adhere Less to the Model

While staff indicated that past related experience improves capability to function and thus improves retention, it can also reduce adherence. Staff with prior clinical experience are sometimes less adherent to the model of care because they wish to practice as they did in prior positions (for example, traditional therapy sessions), and this leads to reduced retention. Another element that determines the level of adherence to the model is patient need for BH—the higher the patient need, the more likely the care teams will step outside the model to satisfy those needs (Figure 3.6).

Figure 3.6
Factors Informing Adherence to the PCBH Model of Care

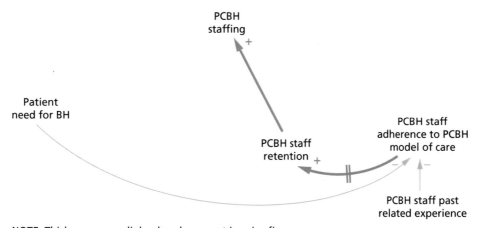

NOTE: Thick arrows are links already present in prior figures.

PCBH Staff Choose to Stay When They Feel More Capable in Their Current PCBH Role, Which Can Take Time to Develop

When PCBH staff feel capable in their current role, that leads to staff satisfaction and, in turn, to retention. Over time, as they do their jobs under engaged program leadership, PCBH staff become more capable of fulfilling their roles in the PCBH program (Figure 3.7). One BHC noted that

Figure 3.7
A Capable, Happy
Workforce Builds Itself

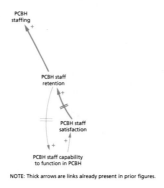

NOTE: Thick arrows are links already present in prior figures.

For probably the first six months to a year, I struggled because I was always behind; I was always seeing patients way too long.

The longer PCBH staff stay, the more time they have to develop capabilities that help them function effectively in the PCBH program. In turn, capability contributes to being satisfied with their jobs in a virtuous cycle that supports staff staying in the position.

Hiring PCBH Staff with More PCBH-Relevant Capabilities as New Hires Makes Them More Capable to Function in PCBH

The better the match between new hires and their roles, the more comfortable they feel in their jobs because they have more of the capabilities that they need from the outset. This, in turn, increases staff satisfaction, which results in increased retention (Figure 3.8).

Figure 3.8
Factors Informing PCBH Staff Capabilities as New Hires

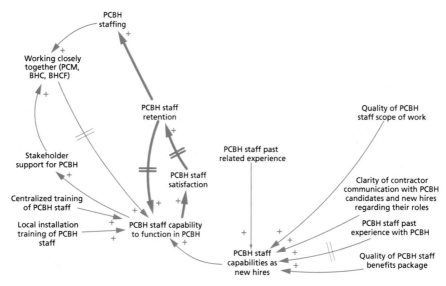

NOTE: Thick arrows are links already present in prior figures.

Several factors affected new hires' level of capability: their own past experience with PCBH, their other past related experience, the clarity of communication of the role (especially with contractors), and the quality of the benefits package.

Other factors influenced existing staff members' level of capability: centralized training, local installation training, and working closely together. There are numerous reinforcing processes here, building over time. For example, when stakeholders (in this case, primary care staff) work more closely together with PCBH staff, staff become more capable, further building support. Also, when staffing is more stable, teamwork builds even more capabilities because teams can work together longer.

Earlier, we mentioned that adequate staffing is not just about the *right level* of staffing. Here, we emphasized having *the right kind of staff*—meaning staff with the right capabilities who enjoy working in this unique type of model and setting.

Retention Is Affected by Understanding of What the Position Entails and Changes in Benefits

Local leadership can work to improve retention by improving the job description. Engaged leaders were able to attract and select new hires who were a good fit by using the improved job descriptions to effectively communicate those role descriptions and expectations during the hiring process (Figure 3.9).

Figure 3.9
A Quality Job Description and Benefits Package Are Useful for Clear Communication to Find the Right Candidates

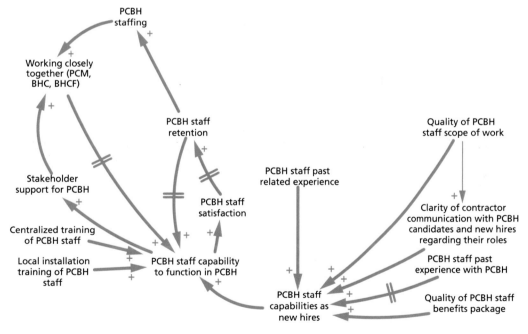

NOTE: Thick arrows are links already present in prior figures.

Participants reported that when this did not happen, new hires were caught by surprise. As one BHCF put it:

> When I got here and found out it was telehealth work and I'd be on the phone all the time, that was a little . . . well, I was disappointed. Let's put it that way.

Lack of understanding of what the position entails is especially common in the context of PCBH staff being hired by contracting organizations, but some staff in GS positions reported lack of understanding of nonclinical responsibilities.

Using Contracting Organizations Instead of GS Staffing Offers Important Advantages and Disadvantages

Important advantages and disadvantages to using contracting organizations instead of GS staffing are displayed in Figure 3.10.

Figure 3.10
Advantages and Disadvantages of Hiring PCBH Staff as GS

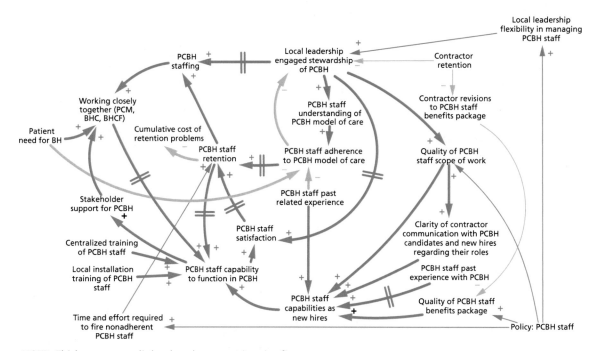

NOTE: Thick arrows are links already present in prior figures.

When contracting organizations are used, employee contracts are regularly renegotiated (often reducing benefits) because the contracting agencies are being bought out before the contract term is up. A PCM, a local leader, and a BHC share some of the disadvantages brought about by having contracting organizations rather than GS positions. A PCM observed,

> Every time the contract is up for renegotiation, you lose some good people.

A local leader offered this perspective:

> They both came to me just so irritated and frustrated [that] they have to reapply for their own jobs. . . . BHCFs had to take a pay cut. I think the BHCs did too. . . . If you want to

keep somebody who's supposed to be embedded in . . . your clinic, you might want to treat them appropriately.

One BHC described a recent experience:

I have [been here] not even two full years . . ., [and] I've had four contract companies . . . because [of] the constant buyouts. . . . It's just so silly. . . . It adds a huge amount of stress . . . because then we have to negotiate [everything] again. . . . Our [paid time off] got slashed this last time, and nobody's happy about that. . . . It's like: "Really? Can we just have a job where it's consistent? Where we know what to expect?" . . . I just wanted to do my job.

Another disadvantage of using contractor organizations is that churning through contractors requires local leadership to spend more time managing the hiring process. Many participants mentioned that a way to improve retention would be to improve the benefits by doing away with the contract renegotiations—for example, by converting the roles to GS positions.

Participants reported that when staff were GS, they had a lot more management tools; participants reported a clear chain of command for monitoring staff, increased flexibility to change work location and hours, more management tools for incentives and rewards, decreased turnover, and increased ability to attract quality applicants. However, participants also reported that they perceived added time and effort required to fire nonadherent staff, something that they identified as contributing to the cumulative cost of retention problems.

Valued Tasks

The Care PCBH Patients Receive Depends on PCM Referrals, Access to PCBH, and the Degree to Which PCMS Work Closely with BHCs and BHCFs

Staff reported that when PCMs, BHCs, and BHCFs work closely together, they do more for their patients.

PCBH patient care tasks are most frequently generated from referrals. Referrals are made by PCMs, but the number and type of referrals depends on the breadth of issues referred to PCBH instead of kept by the PCM or referred to specialty mental health. This depends on what each PCM feels comfortable referring (their level of support).

Accessible BHCs and BHCFs also result in increased patient care, for example, if BHCs and BHCFs are available for PCMs who identify a need for BH during a patient visit to then walk the patient over and make warm introductions for their patient and a BHC or BHCF (i.e., a warm handoff).

PCMs decide the extent to which they engage with each PCBH staff member, but this is limited by the PCBH staff member's resilience. *Resilience* describes the capacity to adapt or change, to keep pace with evolving demands. In the primary care literature, this concept is referred to as *adaptive reserve* (Nutting et al., 2009; Miller et al., 2010; Jaén and Palmer 2012). When PCBH staff resilience is low, PCBH staff are less able to work closely together with PCMs in delivering PCBH care. All of these PCBH patient care tasks contribute to the PCBH staff workload (Figure 3.11).

Figure 3.11
Factors Informing the Amount of PCBH Patient Care

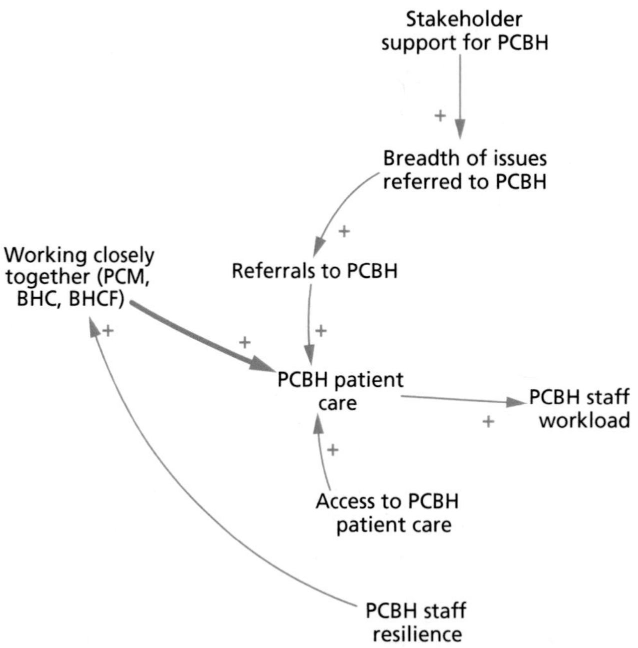

NOTE: Thick arrows are links already present in prior figures.

PCBH Patient Care Tasks Are Central but Not the Only Tasks That Contribute to PCBH Staff Workload

Participants identified various types of patient care tasks as contributing to PCBH workload, such as bridging patient care between primary care and specialty, crisis counseling, providing BH consultation to other staff, group classes, and population health management. They also identified screening,[1] fostering awareness of PCBH, and charting and documenting as important tasks that take time and thus contribute to their workload (see the list of tasks valued by local installation personnel below and Figure 3.12).

- Patient care tasks
  - Bridging patient care between PC and specialty
  - Crisis counseling
  - Providing BH consultation to other staff
  - Group classes
  - Population health management
- Screening
- Fostering awareness of the PCBH program
- Charting and documentation.

---

[1]   The PCBH program design does not call for PCBH staff to do screening except when directly indicated as part of patient care; nevertheless, some participants indicated that PCBH staff are asked to screen patients, even in cases when the screening is also already being done by a primary care staff member.

Figure 3.12
PCBH Staff Workload Is More Than Just Patient Care

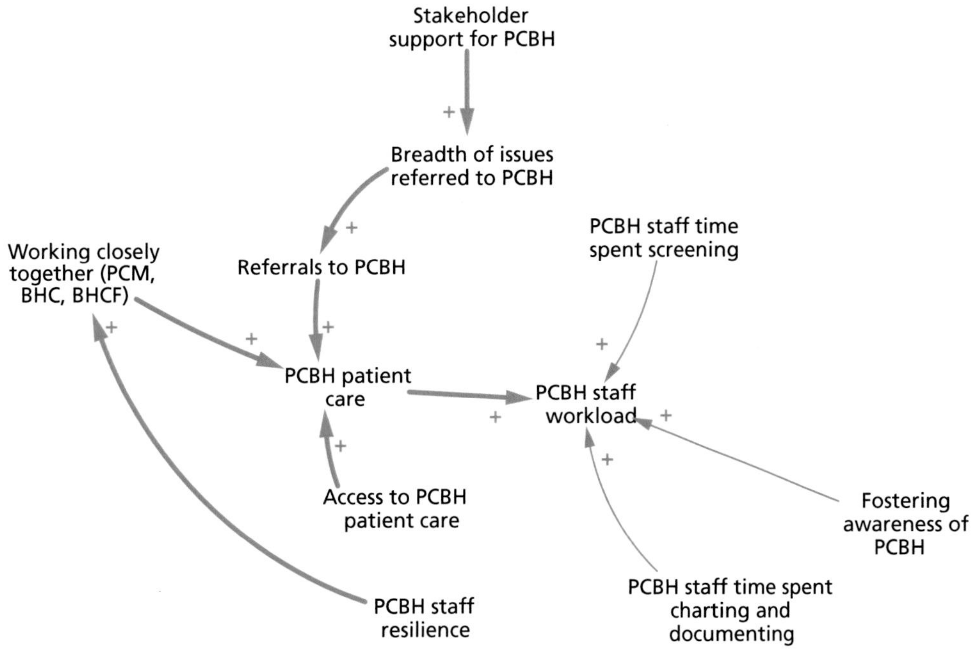

NOTE: Thick arrows are links already present in prior figures.

These additional tasks are important because they enable PCBH staff to address patient needs more fully, to get credit for patient care delivered, and to build support among primary care staff for the PCBH program. More-supportive primary care staff will have a higher breadth of issues that they refer to PCBH staff. Nevertheless, developing and maintaining support among primary care staff requires PCBH staff and local leaders to work at fostering awareness of what PCBH entails and of its value (see the subsequent section on "Fostering PCBH Awareness and Support"). A local leader recounted how this task can sometimes require daily, persistent efforts:

> We tell them [BHCs] to go to the morning huddle. [. . .] Do everything you can to stop by and let them know what you do.

When Workload Becomes Overwhelming, the Care Team Has Ways of Quickly Pushing Back
We found two types of responses that care teams reported using when workload becomes overwhelming: quick responses (described in this section) and others slower to manifest (described in the following two sections).

Teams can quickly push back in various ways (pink arrows in Figure 3.13). BHCs can ask PCMs not to refer so much, or they can limit access to PCBH services by, for example, not being easily available for warm handoffs. Also, they can spend less time on charting and documenting by not documenting everything that they do—but this has unintended consequences for monitoring program performance which is currently focused on number of visits and duration of visits (see "Local leaders can also act as stewards" section below). A BHC reported,

Figure 3.13
Short-Term Pushback to Extreme Workload

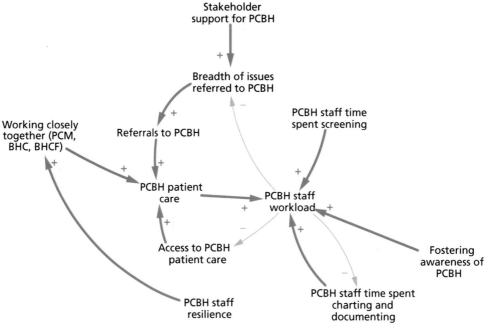

NOTE: Thick arrows are links already present in prior figures.

If I did a note on everybody that I saw with the format we're supposed to I'd be here till nine o'clock.

Shifting to more group visits is conceivable, but such a shift was not mentioned by participants as a viable option for reducing workload because group visits are not incentivized by the current performance metrics.

If the Care Team Cannot Quickly Address Workload Overages, Members Get Burned Out, Corroding Teamwork

Over time, PCBH staff push back in other ways. *A high workload can also have an impact on staff at the individual level, beyond their short-term compensation strategies.* If short-term strategies do not work, staff may begin resisting doing more in PCBH in general. As their resilience decreases, PCBH staff and PCMs start to withdraw from their close working relationships (Figure 3.14).

If That Does Not Work, PCBH Staff May Eventually Quit

Another long-term consequence of workloads that are unsustainable is that they cause PCBH staff to consider quitting. This sets up a slippery slope that makes it harder on everyone who stays, as fewer people share the workload (see new feedback loop in Figure 3.15).

Requesting additional PCBH staff is conceivable but was not mentioned by participants as a viable option for reducing workload. This is because participants reported being under the impression that they needed to meet current performance objectives with current staffing levels, or else they would be at risk of losing existing PCBH staff (and requests for additional

Figure 3.14
Longer-Term Pushback to Extreme Workload

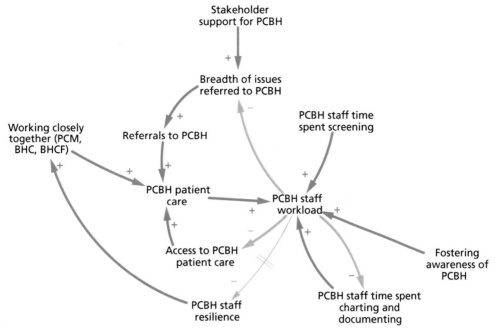

NOTE: Thick arrows are links already present in prior figures.

Figure 3.15
Slippery Slope When Extreme Workload Causes PCBH Staff Retention Problems

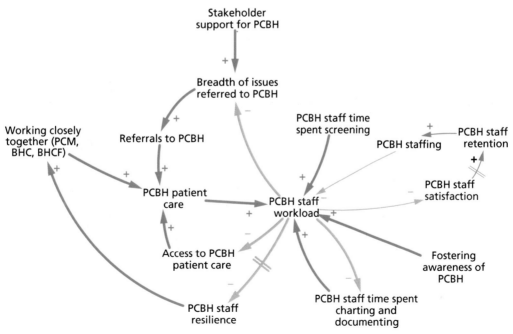

NOTE: Thick arrows are links already present in prior figures.

PCBH staff would be rejected, as they appeared to be unwarranted according to current performance objectives).

PCBH Stewardship

Local Leaders Can Act as Stewards of the PCBH Program by Maintaining Adequate PCBH Staffing Levels and Capability in Four Different Ways

Local leaders with the potential to engage in PCBH stewardship are personnel at the installation in formal or informal leadership roles that touch the PCBH program in some way. Roles identified in interviews include the (informal) BHC or BHCF mentor or trainer for other BHCs and BHCFs at the installation, the OIC at a clinic and other clinic-level local leaders, and the PCBH lead at the installation.

Previous sections identified some ways in which local leaders can act as stewards of the PCBH program by maintaining adequate PCBH staffing levels and capability (see Figure 3.16). These stewardship functions are

Figure 3.16
Local Leadership Stewardship—Monitoring and Action Part 1: Review

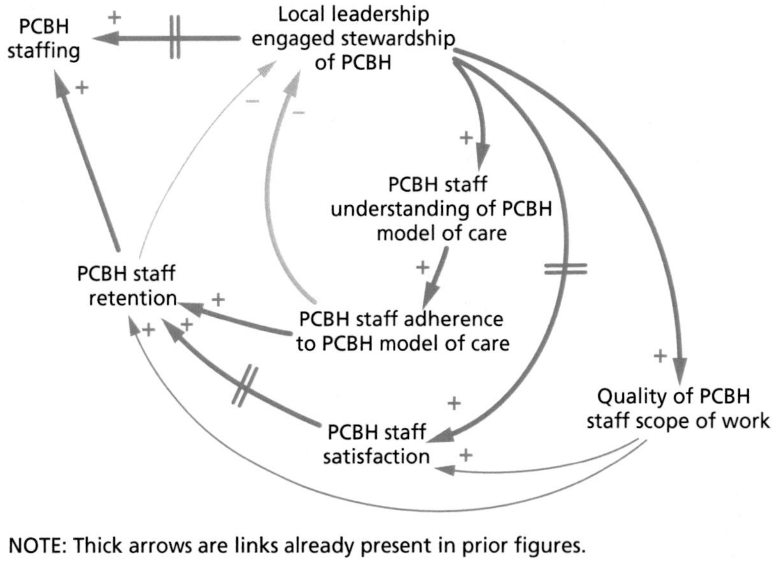

NOTE: Thick arrows are links already present in prior figures.

- hiring new PCBH staff when needed
- working to improve the quality of the scope of work where applicable, which improves PCBH staff satisfaction and retention
- being good managers (which improves PCBH staff satisfaction)—with such habits as making the rounds, explaining policy changes, and investing in process improvement activities
- working with PCBH staff to improve their understanding of the PCBH model of care.

To decide how well they steward the program at any one point in time, engaged local leaders monitor the level of adherence to the PCBH model of care and PCBH staff retention (pink arrows in Figure 3.16).

Local Leaders Can Also Act as Stewards of the PCBH Program by Fostering Awareness

Fostering awareness among installation stakeholders is another way in which local leaders can act as stewards of the PCBH program. Stakeholders are *fully* aware of the PCBH program when their understanding goes beyond individual elements of the program to a comprehensive grasp of how to help patients access it at their installation and the full extent of the value that PCBH can provide. Developing this understanding takes persistence (see "Fostering PCBH Awareness and Support" section below). One local leader opined,

> There [are] a couple clinics that have no idea what to do with a BHCF.

Building awareness increases the chances that stakeholders will support the program. One key stakeholder is the primary care staff, especially PCMs. Each of the local leaders has their own ways of fostering awareness; for example, the PCBH lead at an installation sending their best BHC or BHCF to a clinic where PCBH is not being implemented. Leaders can gauge how much of this work they need to do according to their reading of the current level of support for the program among key stakeholders (see Figure 3.17).

**Figure 3.17
Local Leadership Stewardship—Monitoring
and Action Part 2: Awareness**

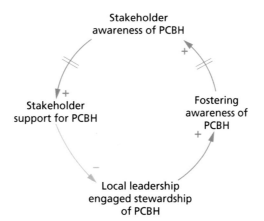

Local Leaders Can Also Act as Stewards by Setting and Monitoring Performance Goals and by Applying Pressure to Meet Those Goals

Local goals are influenced by DHA policies. One way to improve performance is to put pressure on PCMs to refer patients to PCBH. PCMs respond by increasing the breadth of issues that they refer to PCBH, thus increasing referrals to PCBH. By doing so, PCMs reduce the proportion of BH patient needs that they refer to specialty mental health and the proportion of BH patient needs that PCMs address themselves. By reducing their specialty referrals, PCMs are lightening the specialty mental health workload. This should improve access to specialty care. Participants reported that they use PCBH as a bridge to specialty mental health because of experiences with patients unable to access timely specialty mental health care. PCBH staff know the performance objective and respond to shortfalls by increasing access and feeling pressure to increase volume. All of these things influence the volume of patient care. Local leaders update their perceptions of the shortfall between current patient care and performance objectives and reacts accordingly—thus closing these feedback loops (see Figure 3.18).

Figure 3.18
Local Leadership Stewardship—Monitoring and Action Part 3: Performance Objectives

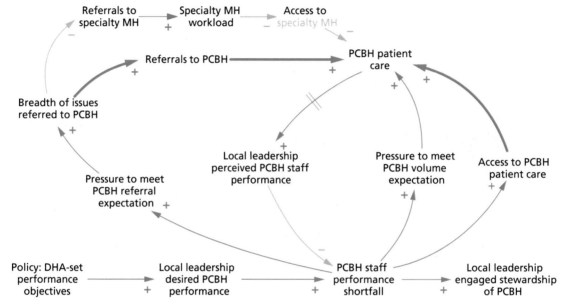

NOTES: Thick arrows are links already present in prior figures. MH = mental health.

The route of all of these loops through patient care reflects staff perceptions that performance objectives are currently focused on number of visits and duration of visits—local PCBH staff tend to express a narrow view of what the job is about. Other tasks, such as the ones identified in Table 2.2, are not visible in performance metrics that staff describe local leaders using to judge program success.

Those in Charge May Not Always Know What They Can Do to Strengthen PCBH

Participants routinely reported that local leaders too often have a narrow understanding of what their role is with respect to PCBH. This section has presented all the ways, identified by participants, in which local leaders have the opportunity to act as stewards of the PCBH program. Figure 3.19 reports what participants identified as the things that engaged local leaders monitor (arrows pointing *toward* "Local leadership engaged stewardship of PCBH") and their subsequent actions (arrows pointing *away from* "Local leadership engaged stewardship of PCBH"). As asserted by participants and visually represented in this figure, monitoring performance (blue box) is just one of local leaders' stewardship roles.

Participants also warned that turnover in local leaders is a concern, given their central role to play in supporting the PCBH program. Participants expressed the concern that new leaders

Figure 3.19
Local Leadership Monitor and Act to Support the PCBH Program

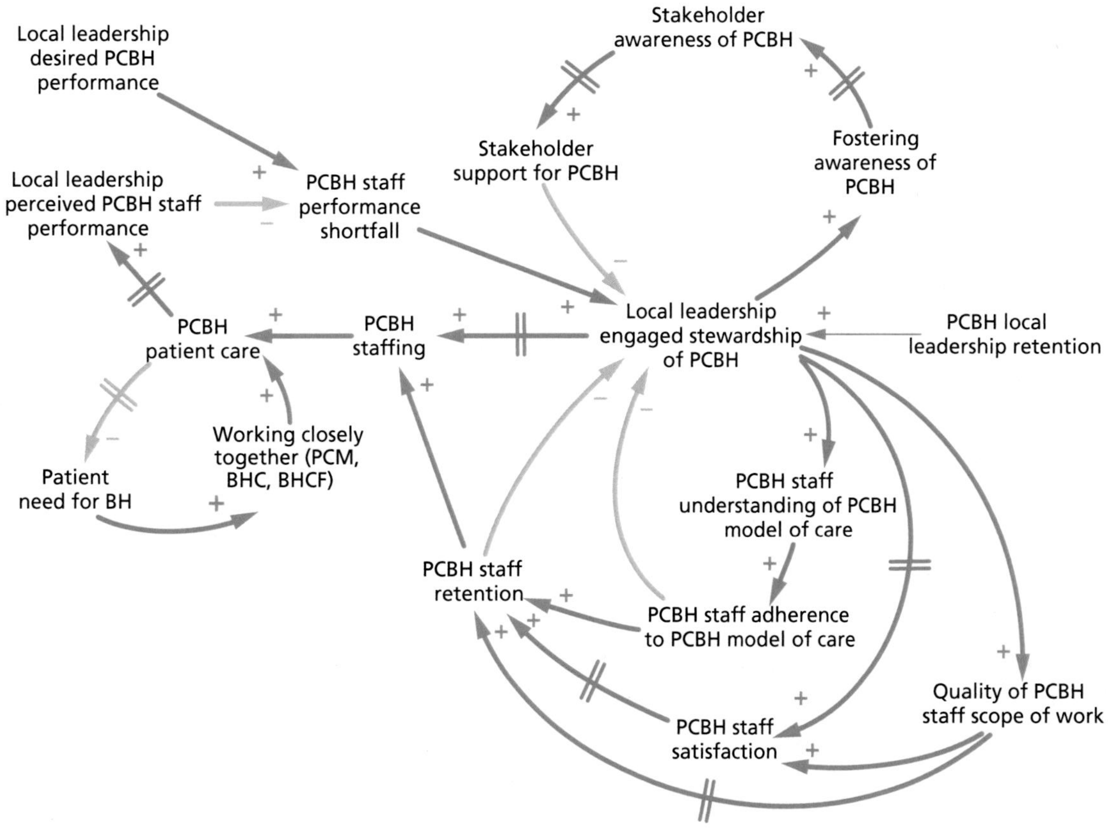

NOTE: Thick arrows are links already present in prior figures.

do not always know or act on all that they can do to strengthen PCBH—or even do all that past leaders at the installation did. As one administrator put it:

> What isn't codified in it is collateral.

Fostering PCBH Awareness and Support

PCBH Success Relies on Supportive Stakeholders

Supportive stakeholders are the foundation of PCBH success (Figure 3.20). Participants reported that unsupportive patients did not come to their appointments. They also reported that unsupportive PCMs did not refer their patients to PCBH—or if they did, under performance pressure, that was only a fraction of the breadth of care that the model is capable of delivering. Participants also reported that unsupportive PCMs were less likely to engage PCBH staff in the teamwork that makes PCBH work as designed.

Participants reported that the support of other stakeholders was also helpful in fostering broad support for the PCBH program. Just as local leaders foster awareness of PCBH, other supportive stakeholders fostered awareness among their peers and others. For example, partici-

Figure 3.20
Impacts of Supportive Stakeholders

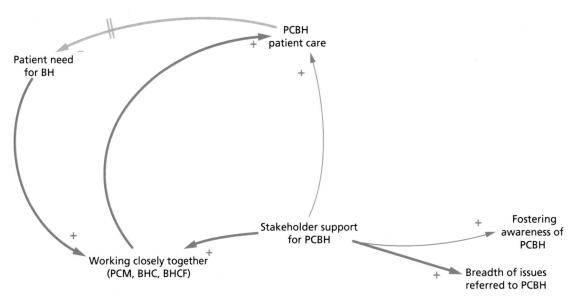

NOTE: Thick arrows are links already present in prior figures.

pants mentioned other stakeholders involved in mental health both in and outside the installation such as chaplains, community groups, and specialty mental health as playing important roles. When supportive, these stakeholders found ways to help the PCBH program, as described by one participant, to break through the "log jam with these with referrals that just weren't making it to [PCBH] behavioral health."

Stakeholders Buy In to PCBH When They Are Fully Aware of the Program and Can See That It Works

As PCBH patient care is delivered, stakeholders perceive that it is working and provide their support (Figure 3.21). For example, PCMs observe that patients are receiving care, and installation leaders see the performance metrics that justify the PCM position. PCMs also become more supportive as they work closely together with PCBH staff because they build routines of cooperation and begin to trust PCBH staff more. Over time, teamwork provides on-the-job training needed by PCBH staff to build the capabilities that further reinforce PCM support. PCMs are also more supportive as they see that PCBH makes them more efficient, that their patients are happy, and that the program has DHA support. In all these ways, PCMs and other local stakeholders are supportive when they see PCBH working well. With respect to perceived performance and patient satisfaction, PCMs remain supportive when they feel confident that the program will provide continuous service to their patients. A gap in service from staff turnover can cause PCMs to lose support.

Stakeholders' pasts also influence their level of support for PCBH. When stakeholders have seen it working well at a prior assignment, they are more supportive. Some stakeholders are just plain cautious about PCBH, even when they see it working around them.

Finally, stakeholders are more supportive of PCBH the more they understand the various aspects of the model. The high rate of turnover among all types of stakeholders at installations

Figure 3.21
Building Supportive Stakeholders

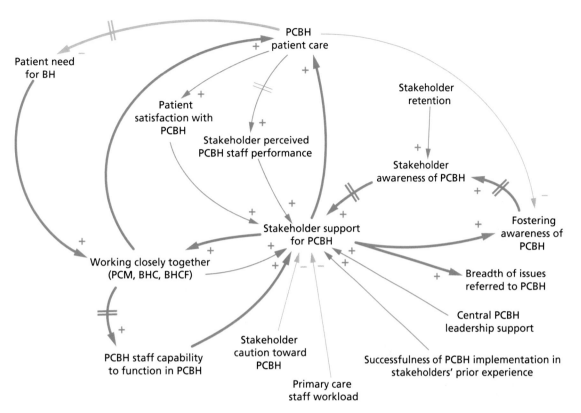

NOTE: Thick arrows are links already present in prior figures.

is detrimental to awareness, necessitating that it be continually attended to. Several stakeholders, including BHCs and BHCFs, will monitor the amount of PCBH patient care being delivered, and when it is low they go out and promote the program to foster awareness. PCBH staff engaging in *routine* promotion works best, especially when such promotion is part of the day-to-day workflow.

Many participants showed a lack of awareness of the BHCF's role. This may be because BHCFs sometimes work in isolation from other staff (screening, scheduling patients), so it is particularly important that they make PCMs and BHCs aware of their role and capabilities. Otherwise, they may risk being ignored or marginalized.

PCMs Are Cross-Cutting Partners in PCBH Implementation

PCMs Play a Role in All Areas of PCBH Implementation

Participants identified PCMs as important players in PCBH implementation. The previous sections each discuss ways in which PCMs contribute to PCBH success. Here we review PCM contributions in each of these areas, and Figure 3.22 presents a visualization.

Figure 3.22
Focusing on PCMs and PCBH (Review)

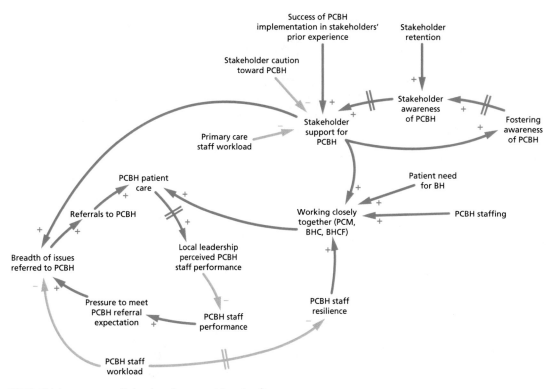

NOTE: Thick arrows are links already present in prior figures.

- **The core of the PCBH program:** PCMs are part of the core of PCBH, given that they choose the extent to which they work closely with PCBH staff in meeting patients' BH needs.
- **PCBH staffing and PCBH capabilities:** PCMs work closely with PCBH staff when they see a need among their patients, and when they have an adequate number of PCBH staff to work with.
- **Valued tasks:** PCMs exercise their judgment and expertise in two areas: (1) how closely they choose to work with PCBH staff members and (2) how broad an array of issues they choose to refer to PCBH staff members. Their choices in both areas affect the level and types of tasks that PCBH staff members perform. An important feedback here is that when the PCBH workload gets overwhelmingly high, PCBH staff are not able to work as closely with PCMs, even when PCMs would continue choosing to work closely with them. Thus, as working closely together increases the PCBH workload, this workload limits the ability to continue working as closely together.
- **PCBH stewardship:** PCMs determine the extent to which they respond to local leadership pressure to increase referrals to PCBH.
- **Fostering PCBH awareness and support:** PCMs are a primary stakeholder in the effort to foster awareness and support—their support enables PCBH to function. PCMs' awareness is influenced by retention; high turnover means a PCM workforce less aware of PCBH. PCMs' willingness to become supportive is influenced by their prior experience

with and caution toward BH in primary care. Supportive PCMs *join with* local leadership and PCBH staff to also foster awareness in their patients and among their colleagues.

PCMs Consider the Impacts of PCBH on Their Own Workload and on Their Patients' Behavioral Health Needs

PCBH staff tasks are strongly coupled with those of the PCM, such that these choices are part of several reinforcing and balancing feedback processes for PCMs (see thin lines in Figure 3.23). PCBH patient care adds work to PCMs' schedules as it becomes a type of screening that identifies issues for PCMs to follow up on. Without teamwork, this can add to PCMs' backlog, potentially causing them to offload some primary care work onto PCBH. When PCMs are able to cope easily with changing situations (i.e., high primary care staff resilience), they will more readily begin teamwork with PCBH. Otherwise, if PCMs' resilience is low, they will not engage in teamwork with PCBH. As the team (BHC, BHCF, PCM) works together, members share tasks, lessening the impact of working with PCBH on the PCM's workload. This improves the PCM's ability to cope with challenges in the future, further reinforcing teamwork. When PCBH staff engage in teamwork, the need for them to fill in for primary care is reduced.

Figure 3.23
Strong Coupling Between PCBH and PCM Tasks Related to BH

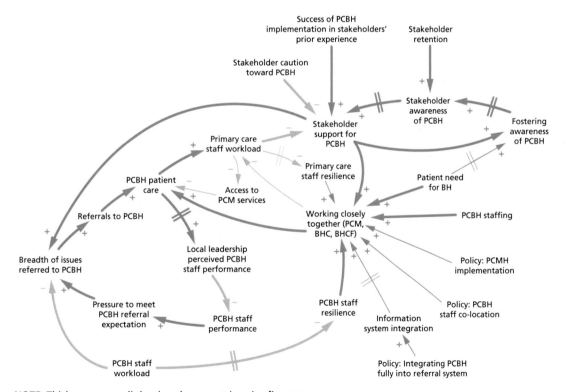

NOTE: Thick arrows are links already present in prior figures.

PCMs are particularly knowledgeable about their patients' need for BH and their patients' awareness of PCBH. As they sense that patients need more BH services, they work to foster awareness of PCBH. This often includes strategic efforts to deal with patients' BH stigma (e.g., warm handoffs to PCBH staff, starting with sleep concerns before addressing deeper issues).

Several policies affect PCMs' ability to work closely with PCBH staff: PCMH implementation, PCBH staff co-location, and full integration of PCBH into PCMs' referral system. Participants reported that PCMH implementation creates care teams that can more easily incorporate PCBH staff. They also reported that co-location in the clinic improves PCMs' ability to develop relationships and communicate well with PCBH staff. Finally, participants noted that current information systems for BH and primary care are not well integrated, so staff use workarounds to improve the situation, and this takes time. Improving such systems would improve staff members' ability to work closely together.

Causal Feedbacks in the PCBH Program

A key purpose of this report is to evaluate the PCBH program by building understanding of the causal feedback loops operating in PCBH across installations and contexts while also communicating what these loops mean for various ongoing PCBH processes. The previous sections presented the majority of these loops found in the interviews. Taken as a whole, these loops visualize the complex nature of the various causes of challenges and successes in PCBH. This section presents this holistic understanding in one comprehensive CLD. Various views are generated to highlight different aspects of this one comprehensive CLD (as in Figures 3.26–3.27 and figures in Appendix C). These views are also available on Kumu:[2] https://RANDCorp. kumu.io/pcbh.

The four topics described earlier are primarily located in specific places on the comprehensive CLD. Figure 3.25 shows this using blue boxes. The blue boxes show that none of these topics is independent of the rest. Each topic area is closely linked with the others via positive and negative feedback loops. In keeping with this interdependency, our recommendations are also cross-cutting—that is, each one addresses multiple related issues.

While all variables are treated the same in the foregoing CLDs, the following comprehensive CLDs use three background colors to distinguish the degree of control stakeholders have and each variable's location in relation to causal feedback loops: gray for context variables that are hard to influence, gray and green for policies under DHA/Program Manager control, yellow for actions under frontline staff direct control; other variables are transparent (see Figure 3.24). Figure 3.26 shows the comprehensive CLD (in Kumu, this is the *decisions, policy, context* view). Figure 3.27 adds loop labels that briefly describe each feedback process (in Kumu, this is the *decisions, policy, context with loop labels* view). In Kumu, each loop label can be selected to show all of the variables and links in that loop.

Shared Understanding Diagrams (in Appendix C) document the level of shared understanding of model contents within a role (BHC, BHCF, PCM, local leaders) and within a service (Air Force, Army, Navy). Diagrams show that the *breadth* of collective perception of PCBH processes and *depth* at which that perception is shared vary across roles and services.

---

[2]   This platform permits users to interact with the diagram and to read it one piece at a time by selecting an element, such as a variable name, link, or loop label. Hovering over an element temporarily highlights the content that is closely linked to it, and the *focus* feature shows this content exclusively and also zooms in on it. Multiple elements can be selected and focused on using the Shift key.

Figure 3.24
Variable Types in Comprehensive CLD

		Is the variable located inside or outside of a causal loop?	
		Inside	Outside
What degree of control do PCBH stakeholders have?	High	Actions under frontline staff direct control	Policies under DHA/Program Manager control
	Low	Other influences	Context variables that are hard to influence

The level of depth is indicated by the thickness of arrows, and the breadth is indicated by the number of thicker arrows. BHCs have the greatest depth and breadth of shared understanding regarding the PCBH program, followed by the local leaders. Earlier, we reported that the BHCF role is less well understood and that some leaders are not planning to hire more BHCFs to replace those that have left. The BHCF Shared Understanding diagram indicates that, while BHCFs recognize that fostering awareness matters for building support and thus implementation, fewer of them mentioned these links in their interviews relative to the proportion of participants mentioning these links in other roles.

Even though stakeholders may have a relatively high degree of control over a variable, they may not necessarily have much control over the consequences and may lack awareness about how their previous actions shape the information that they use in their decisionmaking. This is more likely to be the case for longer feedback loops. These comprehensive CLDs make these loops visible.

Figure 3.25
High-Level Overview—Four Areas of the PCBH Program

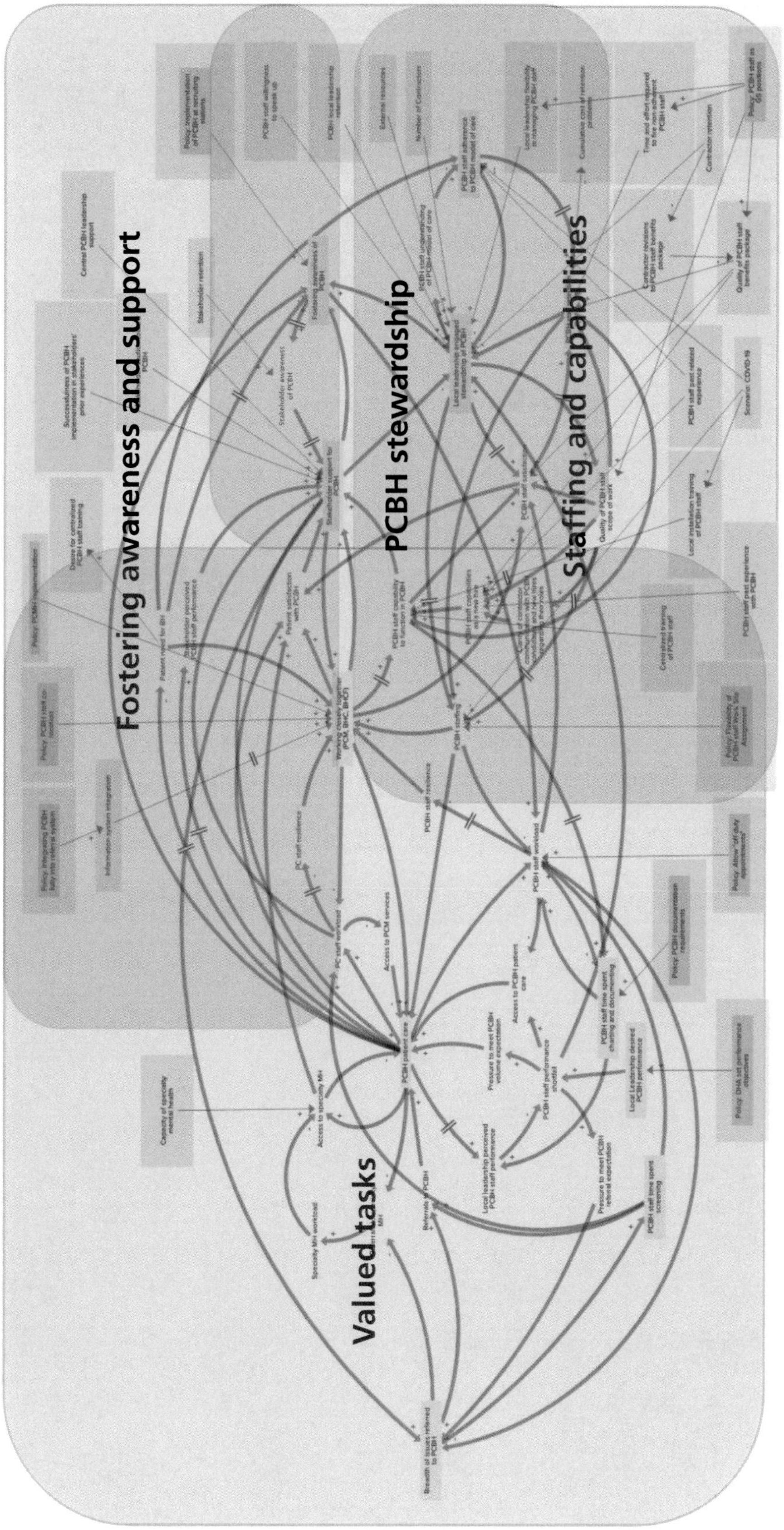

Figure 3.26
PCBH Program Causal Loop Diagram—Without Loop Labels

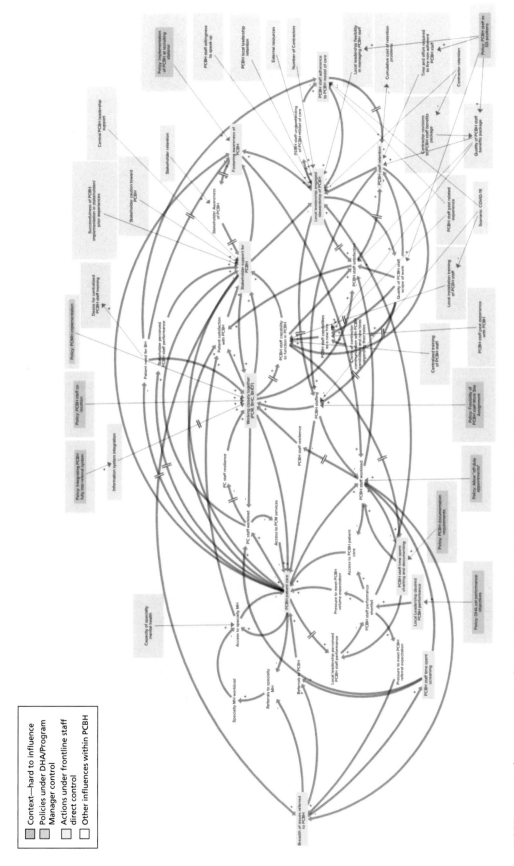

NOTE: In Kumu, https://RANDCorp.kumu.io/pcbh, this is the *decisions, policy, context* view.

Figure 3.27
PCBH Program Causal Loop Diagram—with Loop Labels

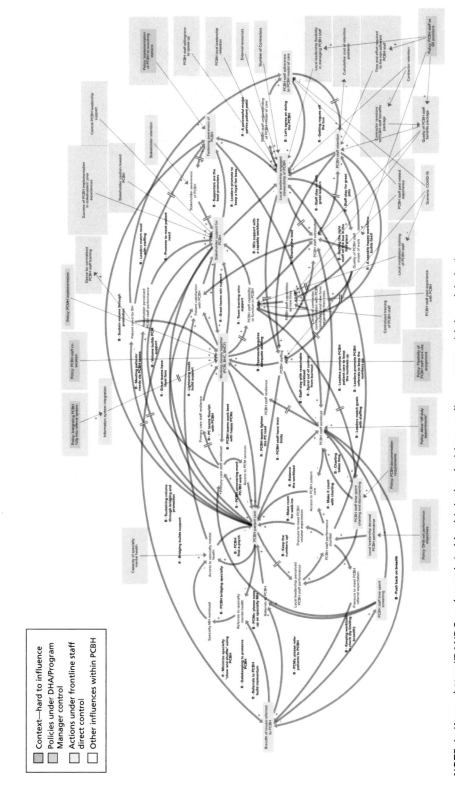

NOTE: In Kumu, https://RANDCorp.kumu.io/pcbh, this is the *decisions, policy, context with loop labels* view.

CHAPTER FOUR

Summary, Conclusions, and Recommendations

Summary of Key Interview Results

PCBH Staffing and Capabilities

Adequate PCBH staffing is crucial to PCBH success. It is important to have appropriate *levels* of staffing, as well as staff with the right *capabilities*. Retention of existing staff is influenced by the quality of benefits and the job description. Contractor benefits are not adequate to maintain capable staff, given the downward spiral with renegotiated contracts. Job descriptions are also inadequate for identifying candidates whose interests and skills match the positions, and for helping the candidates to know what to expect in the role. When PCBH staff do have the right capabilities, PCMs work more closely with them—and working together, in turn, helps develop these capabilities.

We found that adherence to the brief, consultative PCBH model varies. Sometimes staff do not adhere to the model because patient needs cannot be met within the constraints of the model (e.g., due to a lack of specialty care availability). However, lack of adherence is sometimes due to a desire to practice as they practiced in a previous job.

Valued Tasks

The level of PCBH patient care depends on PCM *willingness to refer* to PCBH and *breadth of issues* that PCMs are willing to refer to PCBH.

Tasks besides patient care keep the program running, but nonclinical tasks have less visibility. Staff manage their workloads by pushing back on less visible tasks, by working less closely with primary care staff, and even by leaving the position if conditions do not improve.

We also found that close teamwork of PCBH staff with primary care staff generates more patient care. This might seem so obvious as to be taken for granted. A PCM who does not closely engage with PCBH staff members will be able to provide only a limited amount of PCBH care because the primary care and PCBH staff members will never work closely enough to develop the capabilities on-the-job to really have the PCM engage with the full breadth of issues that PCBH staff members can offer their patients.

PCBH Stewardship

Local leaders are often found to perform *some but not all* of the stewardship roles reported as valuable—key factors here are turnover and the need for codification of additional valued roles.

Effective local leaders *actively monitor* adherence, performance, support, and retention to inform their level of stewardship.

Fostering PCBH Awareness and Support

Everyone involved has a role to play in promoting awareness of the PCBH program. Fostering program awareness is often seen as the responsibility of BHCs, but program success also relies on PCMs referring for the full breadth of problems that PCBH staff can address, and other stakeholders can also refer to the program. PCMs and other stakeholders buy into PCBH when they are fully aware of the program and can see that it works. Teamwork and understanding of the model help bolster PCM support for PCBH staff, but turnover makes maintaining support more challenging. We found that *routine,* day-to-day promotion of the program works best. However, we note that there is often a particular lack of awareness of the BHCF role.

Causal Feedbacks in the PCBH Program

Taken as a whole, the diagram of feedback loops we have derived from all participants' experiences with PCBH presents a causal explanation for the range of challenges and successes that participants described in engaging with the PCBH program. This holistic understanding is presented in one comprehensive CLD that can express the stories of all participants. It contains context variables that are hard to influence, policies under DHA/Program Manager control, actions under frontline staff direct control, and other influences. Even though stakeholders may have a relatively high degree of control over a variable, they may not necessarily have much control over consequences and may lack awareness about how their previous actions shape the information that they use in their decisionmaking. This is more likely to be the case for longer feedback loops. The comprehensive CLD renders these loops visible and, thus, makes it easier for policymakers to understand varying implementation experiences and to consider program changes in light of both direct consequences and knock-on effects.

Recommendations to Improve Behavioral Health Patient Care Delivered in Primary Care

We present recommendations in the four areas highlighted in our findings: staffing and capabilities, valued tasks, program stewardship, and fostering awareness and support of the program. We discuss each of these in turn. We note that some of the suggested changes can be implemented at the program level, while other recommendations are outside of the program's control and would require higher-level Department of Defense (DoD) intervention to address systemic issues.

PCBH Staffing and Capabilities

Improve job descriptions. Hiring and retaining qualified staff is essential for program success, but the PCBH program is not consistently able to attract staff with the right interests and capabilities. We found that contractors often had a poor understanding of what their positions entailed before commencing work. For example, BHCs were surprised that the position did not entail provision of psychotherapy, and BHCFs were surprised that their roles involved less in-person clinical contact than they assumed. In contrast to contractors, GS PCBH staff typically had a strong up-front understanding of their clinical roles, but they still did not understand their nonclinical duties (e.g., actively advertising their role, working closely with PCMs to increase referrals) until they started work.

Consequently, we recommend that the program improve job descriptions to ensure that applicants have a comprehensive understanding of the positions and can better self-assess whether their skills and interests are a match. We suggest ensuring that job descriptions convey the high volume of clinical work (i.e., large number of brief appointments) and clearly describe nonclinical duties so that staff consider those tasks part of the job. We further suggest encouraging local installation contracting offices to require contracting organizations to accurately convey what the positions entail.

Improve the contracting process and/or transition key PCBH staff positions to GS. Contractor staff reported frequently experiencing changes in salary and/or benefits as a result of contractor buyouts or mergers. Changes in benefits reduced reported staff satisfaction and were cited as a major contributor to staff turnover. Therefore, we recommend improving the contracting process and/or transitioning key PCBH staff positions to GS.

Regarding improvements to contracting, while DHA and the PCBH Program Managers do not have control over contractor salaries and benefits, it may be possible to work with installation contracting offices to **incentivize contracting organizations to reduce turnover**. For instance, it may be possible to bring more installations under a Performance Work Statement and to build economic penalties for lack of retention into the agreement, so that contracting organizations are incentivized to recruit individuals who are a match for the positions and provide them with benefits that make them want to stay. In this scenario, contracting organizations might find it more cost-effective to improve recruitment and provide better benefits than to incur penalties for turnover.

Aside from retention issues, local leaders have expressed that contractors are more difficult to manage than GS staff because of a lack of flexibility in what they can ask of staff. We recommend urging contracting offices to **incorporate management tools into contracts**, including flexibility in work hours, ability to move staff between clinics on the installation or to split staff members' time between clinics, and inclusion of a comprehensive range of tasks so that everything management might ask PCBH staff to do is allowable under the contract.

If it is not possible to improve the contracting process, we recommend **transitioning key PCBH positions to GS**. There are inherent difficulties with a contract approach when seeking a highly specialized workforce, such as that required by the PCBH program. Given the considerable investment in training BHCs in particular, adopting a hiring model that makes it easier to retain valued staff makes sense. The GS model protects the program's investment in staff training and allows provision of professional development, which is not allowed for nongovernment staff. Given GS hiring caps, transitioning key positions to GS may require working to obtain MTF commander buy-in to use available slots for this purpose or higher-level DoD intervention to ensure GS slot availability for PCBH staff.

Prioritize rapid rehiring. We found that when PCBH services are not consistently available, patient access to care is reduced and PCMs are more reluctant to refer to BHCs. Consequently, we recommend prioritizing rapid rehiring after turnover to minimize gaps in service and ensure that the staff role continues to be valued. However, it should be noted that hiring is slow due to factors largely out of the program's control. Indeed, while hiring delays are particularly problematic in this relatively new program, they are a larger, systemic issue likely affecting many DoD programs. Higher-level DoD intervention will therefore be needed to address this issue. DoD should consider reviewing its hiring processes to see what can be done to expedite them. An alternative strategy could be to consider building reserve capacity to mitigate the impact of slow hiring processes.

Valued Tasks

Identify, count, and reinforce valued tasks. In addition to providing patient care in the brief model, BHCs and BHCFs take on many other tasks. Some of these tasks are clearly valued as central to program implementation (e.g., "clinical productivity behaviors" such as PCM outreach). Other tasks may or may not be valued (e.g., providing therapy as a bridge between primary and specialty care, when provision of more intensive services typically causes BHCs to see fewer patients). Although BHC performance criteria acknowledge various domains, productivity looms largest in staff minds on a day-to-day basis.

We recommend identifying all valued tasks and giving them increased visibility, protecting and dedicating time for them, and targeting them in routine, *ongoing* training. Giving credit, time, and support for all valued tasks should result in increased staff satisfaction. In addition, it allows for identification of redundancies that do not add value (e.g., PCM, PCBH, and patient completing screening forms where the patient is asked the same questions multiple times).

Continue to work toward awareness of tasks and roles—beyond BHC. We recommend increasing efforts to promote understanding of the BHCF role and local (clinic and installation) leadership roles. While BHC roles are widely understood, BHCF roles tend to be poorly understood, and thus BHCFs tend to be underutilized in PCBH implementation. Additional attention is needed to ensure that PCMs and the entire care team are aware of the services BHCFs are able to provide.

Since the role of BHCs is largely understood, the techniques that worked well for BHCs can serve as a model for promoting awareness of BHCFs. BHCFs can market themselves in all the ways that successful BHCs currently self-promote (e.g., attending morning huddles, posting and distributing flyers and brochures that explain how they can help, reviewing PCM patient lists, reaching out to providers on a regular basis). BHCs and BHCFs can also partner in promoting the roles that each of them plays. These kinds of BHCF marketing techniques are already working well at some installations but do not currently occur at other sites.

Local leadership roles are also inconsistently understood, and we will discuss our recommendations in detail in the next sections on program stewardship and fostering PCBH awareness. Briefly, we encourage cultivation of local champions and increased orientation and ongoing communication with local leadership regarding their roles. The PCBH program is now holding in-briefs with supervisors after every new BHC onboarding. This is a promising approach that could be expanded to include BHCFs. Beyond that, because there is high turnover in PCMs and local leadership, we suggest also providing orientation after any changes in local PCM and leadership staffing. We recommend that PCM and local leadership orientation include introduction to the BHC and BHCF roles, as well as introduction to their own roles in the PCBH model.

PCBH Stewardship

Effective stewardship of the PCBH program is vital. We have a number of recommendations for enhancing the role of program leadership.

Increase support for local leadership. It is vital to have effective stewardship and support of the program at the clinic and installation leadership levels (e.g., OIC, PCBH champion) so that the burden of program success does not lie so much on the shoulders of individual BHCs. Local primary care leaders have a lot of responsibilities outside of the PCBH program, and as a result, local leaders did not consistently know that much about their roles in the program. To address that, we recommend **increasing orientation and ongoing communication with local leadership** regarding their roles. We suggest encouraging local leadership to level with PCBH staff about expectations and engage with staff on problem-solving early and often (e.g., helping staff manage workload or the low level of referrals from PCMs). We also suggest assisting local leadership in helping BHCs and BHCFs in fostering awareness of the PCBH program—which we will discuss further in the next section. It is important to allow flexibility in how local leaders oversee the program; local PCBH leadership roles should be codified but tailored to local needs.

Implement routine measurement and monitoring of *comprehensive* metrics. We recommend that central program leadership and local installation leadership routinely use a comprehensive set of implementation metrics and performance objectives in assessing how things are going. A comprehensive set of metrics might encompass referrals, workload, BHC and BHCF staffing levels; staff satisfaction and retention; and population health indicators (i.e., patient mental health status across the PCM's panel; such measurement begins with BHCFs using Healthcare Effectiveness Data and Information Set data but continues with recording their sense of the extent to which telehealth patients are getting better). We recommend providing sites with more training on how to use utilization and symptom outcomes measures to monitor patients and the program.

We further suggest **setting "trip wires" that flag the need for action** (e.g., for high or low BHC workload, low BHCF utilization, low PCM referrals, low mental health status across a PCM's panel). We recommend monitoring PCBH metrics and performance objectives both centrally and locally. Locally, we recommend allowing flexibility to tailor oversight, metrics, and objectives to local pressures (e.g., specialty care availability) while still ensuring consistency with the central model.

It will be important to identify whose role it is to monitor these metrics centrally (DHA or Psychological Health Center of Excellence) and, especially, locally (within a clinic or installation).

Less formally, it may be helpful to encourage PCBH staff to speak up to leadership about workload issues so that these issues can be addressed early on, perhaps even before a trip wire is activated.

Cultivate local champions. Indeed, local support for the PCBH program is vital, because it is challenging to manage the program centrally. To this end, we recommend that the PCBH managers increase their efforts to **identify and cultivate installation-level champions**. Different types of staff might serve as local champions, but we suggest that the champion should be a GS to minimize turnover in the role and have greater influence over job descriptions. For instance, one BHC per installation could be a GS with core responsibilities that include monitoring metrics, contract stewardship and oversight, and fostering awareness of the program. In this way, there would be enhanced local support for implementing our recommendations around improving contracting, monitoring metrics, and fostering program awareness (discussed in the next section). The local champion's job description would ideally tie their job performance to performance of the program as a whole.

Increase central support for local PCBH staff. BHCs spoke favorably of the training provided but often still did not feel comfortable treating the full breadth of conditions intended to be treated by the model. We recommend efforts to **continuously build BHC skills** so that they are comfortable treating the full range of conditions, and PCMs are comfortable referring for the full breadth of conditions. The program can periodically advertise available training resources, such as the webinars accessible on the PCBH website. Central program leadership can also curate an approved list of outside trainings that BHCs can participate in and advertise these trainings along with internally developed webinars. Because BHCs vary in their comfort in treating different conditions in the brief model, we recommend that each BHC develop and implement a personalized plan for skill development. We further recommend that BHCs be provided with protected time for completing training, potentially with a requirement to complete a personal skill development plan.

We recommend provision of **regular, ongoing support for BHCs and BHCFs.** One key way to do this is through monthly calls. BHCs appreciated these calls when they occurred, and they were recently reinstated. In addition to program managers providing support for local PCBH staff, local staff can use the calls to inform central leadership regarding what is going on on the ground (e.g., changes in local leadership or other local context for PCBH program implementation).

We further recommend **more ongoing orientation for PCMs** regarding PCBH and their role in the program, including how to work closely with BHCs and BHCFs. In particular, we suggest **providing more orientation to the BHCF role and how it adds value**.

Fostering PCBH Awareness and Support

Provide more central assistance in fostering awareness of the PCBH program. BHCs play a key role in fostering awareness of PCBH, but responsibility for program promotion and, thus, success can be shared among more staff. We recommend increasing support for local leadership in routinely promoting close teamwork and awareness of PCBH. For instance, as described in the stewardship section above, orientation for local leadership can play a critical role. We also suggest that central PCBH leadership can provide ongoing guidance to local leadership in implementation of routine application and monitoring of implementation and performance metrics. Because engagement of local leadership can be challenging, we suggest periodic video meetings that focus on collaborative problem-solving with a small group of installations instead of more frequent, larger leadership meetings.

We further recommend that central program leadership **do more to promote awareness of the BHCF role**. As described in the valued tasks section, the same strategies that effectively promote awareness of BHCs can be used to promote awareness of BHCFs. For instance, any centrally developed promotional materials, orientation, communication, and outreach strategies used to promote BHC awareness can also be used for BHCFs. Ideally, there would be versions of materials that promote the BHC and BHCF together as complementary parts of the PCBH treatment team.

Some installations are locally developing promotional materials, suggesting that they are unaware of centrally developed materials and/or that the available materials do not fully meet their needs. In response, we suggest **regularly updating and disseminating** centrally developed promotional materials for both BHC and BHCF services. Materials already generated at the local level can be reviewed and added to the materials repository.

Conclusions

This analysis has identified a number of important facilitators and challenges in the implementation of PCBH and made clear the complex, interdependent ways in which they are linked.

This improved understanding opens up a great opportunity for DHA to have a meaningful impact on the integration of BH into primary care and thus on patient health. DHA can also use this understanding to inform local installation PCBH stakeholders on best practices that they can adopt for implementing the program in their context.

Study participants across a broad range of stakeholder groups attested to the unique and important role that PCBH can and sometimes does play in addressing patients' BH needs. The PCBH program is highly valued by primary care staff when it works well at meeting patient need. The PCBH model is inconsistently adhered to owing to a combination of staff preferences, local pressures, and lack of awareness of PCBH staff roles. There is great opportunity for this program to have a meaningful impact on service members' health and wellbeing. Participants noted that DHA has influence over important aspects, such as performance objectives and codification of PCBH-related local leadership and staff roles.

However, the success of this program is beyond the control of any single stakeholder group. Our research also makes clear the important roles that local leaders, PCMs, BHCs and BHCFs can have in determining a clinic's journey through PCBH implementation. Our research found that local stakeholders' actions are tied up in numerous feedback loops. These became visible as individuals' perspectives were merged into one comprehensive diagram. As long as these feedbacks remain largely invisible to local PCBH stakeholders, the potential for unintended consequences remains high.

The research also has revealed opportunities to improve approaches toward PCBH implementation and leads to recommendations specific to PCBH staffing and capabilities, valued tasks, stewardship, and fostering awareness and support.

By mapping the causal links expressed in a wide array of PCBH experiences across installations into one CLD, this study has identified a number of important facilitators and challenges at play in the Air Force, Army, and Navy. Overall, the research team has built understanding of the causal feedback loops between policies and stakeholder actions operating in PCBH across installations and contexts while also communicating what these loops mean for various ongoing PCBH processes. The results of the study provide an evidence-based understanding of the facilitators of and challenges to delivering BH care services to service members using the PCBH program model of care, an understanding that policymakers can use in shaping the future of the PCBH program.

PCBH Logic Model

The RAND team developed the PCBH Logic Model collaboratively, with input from the program managers in charge of PCBH implementation, the PCBH program developers, and DCoE staff members. This Logic Model was used to inform the development of evaluation questions and, consequently, data collection instruments. Figure A.1 is a visual representation of the PCBH Logic Model.

**Figure A.1
The PCBH Logic Model**

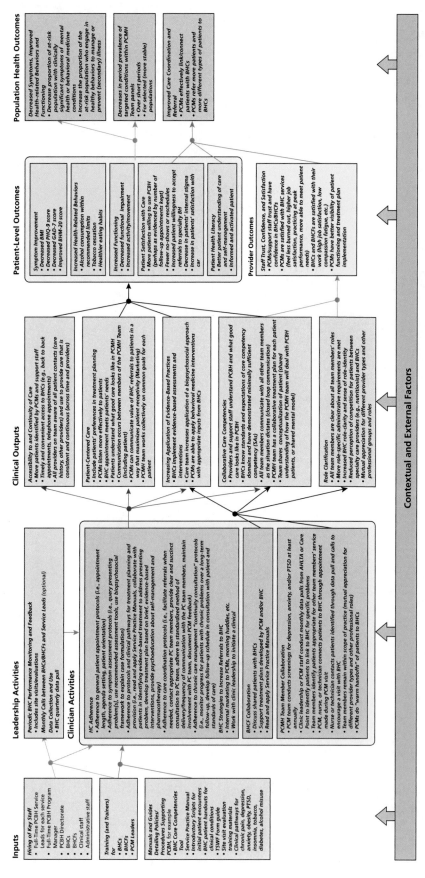

NOTE: 5As = five major steps to intervention; AHLTA = Armed Forces Health Longitudinal Technology Application; BHM-20 = Behavioral Health Measure 20; BMI = body-mass index; GAD-7 = General Anxiety Disorder 7-question diagnostic test; TSWF = Tri-Service Work Flow; PC = primary care; PHQ-9 = Patient Health Questionnaire 9.

Example of a Rigorously Coded and Interpreted Quotation

Interview transcripts were rigorously coded to identify the variables and causal links inside the stories that participants shared. The evaluation team went through iterative rounds of coding that began with identifying causal language in the text data. We developed a coding scheme using interviews from one installation and refined it as needed as new concepts arose in coding data from additional installations. This coding scheme did more than just identify elements: Excerpts of causal language were converted into simple CLD-type word and arrow diagrams to identify the variable being discussed and to signify the direction in which causality flows. Figure B.1 is an example of this type of coding.

Figure B.1
Sample Coded Quotation from a Participant Interview

Quotation
C-R1-1-A-1-05: "You know, I know that was a huge thing in my civilian life where I would refer people to psych either they would never get scheduled or there was a six-month wait period and folks would just give up but when I was working in a clinic where I had a behavioral health person and could do warm handoffs there immediately engaged and in the system so to say so it gives you a better chance of latching onto them and then we have our Behavioral Health Care facilitator who was people who seem to be dropping off she can reach out to them and she reaches out for medication compliance and things like that. So, you know, we have the the sort of full circle here, which is great."

Phrases from the quotation	CLD elements
it gives you a better chance of latching onto them	**Patient need for behavioral health**
people who seem to be dropping off she can reach out to them and she reaches out for medication compliance and things like that	**Patient need for behavioral health**
could do warm handoffs there immediately engaged and in the system so to say so it gives you a better chance of latching onto them and	**Working closely together (PCM, BHC, BHCF)**
could do warm handoffs there immediately engaged and in the system so to say so it gives you a better chance of latching onto them and	**PCBH patient care**
but when I was working in a clinic where I had a behavioral health person and could do warm handoffs there immediately engaged and in the system	**PCBH patient care**
then we have our Behavioral Health Care facilitator who was people who seem to be dropping off she can reach out to them and she reaches out for medication compliance and things like that. So, you know, we have the the sort of full circle here, which is great	**PCBH patient care**
we have the the sort of full circle here, which is great	(Information feedback)

Causal link	Interpretation
Patient need for behavioral health-->+ Working closely together (PCM, BHC, BHCF)	PCM recalls how it was difficult to address patient needs in his civilian practice. In PCBH, this patient need entices him to work with the PCBH staff.
Working closely together (PCM, BHC, BHCF)-->+ PCBH patient care	PCM sends patients to PCBH using "warm handoffs" to help patients who need BH access PCBH care.
PCBH patient care--//-->- Patient need for behavioral health	In addition to "warm handoffs," PCBH provides a comprehensive set of services for patients with behavioral health needs, in particular, the care management role BHCFs play. These services contribute to meeting patient needs – thus coming "full circle."

Shared Understanding Diagrams

Shared Understanding diagrams (Figures C.1–C.7) document the level of shared understanding of model contents within a role (BHC, BHCF, PCM, local leaders) and within a service (Air Force, Army, Navy). These CLDs show that the *breadth* of collective perception of PCBH processes and *depth* at which that perception is shared vary across these groups (roles and services). The level of depth is indicated by the thickness of arrows, and the breadth is indicated by the number of thicker arrows.

These diagrams are also available on Kumu: https://RANDCorp.kumu.io/pcbh. Each diagram can be accessed by selecting a different *view* (the menu of views is located at the top left of the viewing screen). The viewer may then examine the diagram in its entirety or read it one piece at a time by selecting an element, such as a variable name, link, or loop label (see Figure 3.27 in Chapter Three for a version of the overall CLD with loop labels). Hovering over an element temporarily highlights the content that is closely linked to it, and the *focus* feature shows this content exclusively and also zooms in on it. Multiple elements can be selected and focused on by clicking on them using the Shift key.

The primary purpose of these diagrams is to communicate the level of saturation for each link in the comprehensive CLD. These figures identify the links that are most frequently discussed by each group (thick arrows). They also identify the links that are less-often discussed by each group (thin arrows). In so doing, they convey the level of confidence we have about each link. A secondary purpose is to consider variations in understanding across groups. Thick lines show links that are well-understood, while thin lines show darker spots in participants' understanding. When a feedback loop has mixed thick and thin lines, it indicates that it is probably a *dark loop*—a causal feedback process that few people were recognizing. The more dark loops, the more likely that decisions will produce unintended consequences. We do not propose that these diagrams be used for comparison across groups but rather for introspection within groups.

Figure C.1
Shared Understanding—Navy

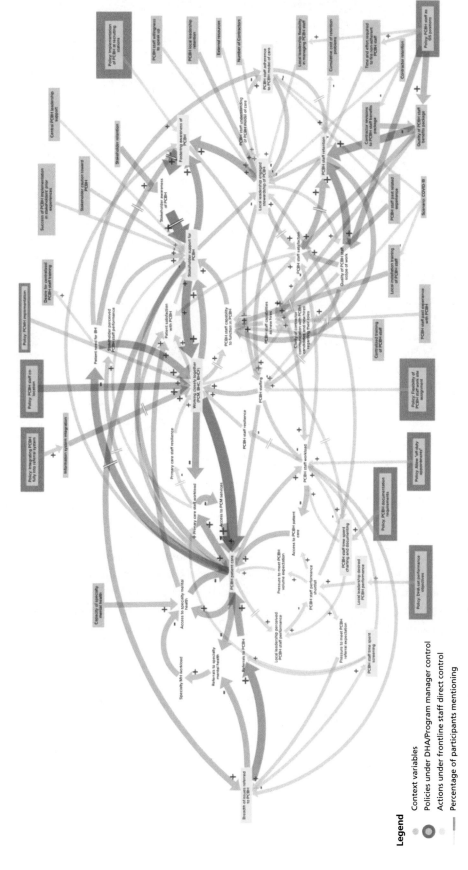

Legend

Context variables
Policies under DHA/Program manager control
Actions under frontline staff direct control
Percentage of participants mentioning

NOTE: In Kumu, https://RANDCorp.kumu.io/pcbh, this is the *Shared Understanding Diagram—Navy* view.

Figure C.2
Shared Understanding—Army

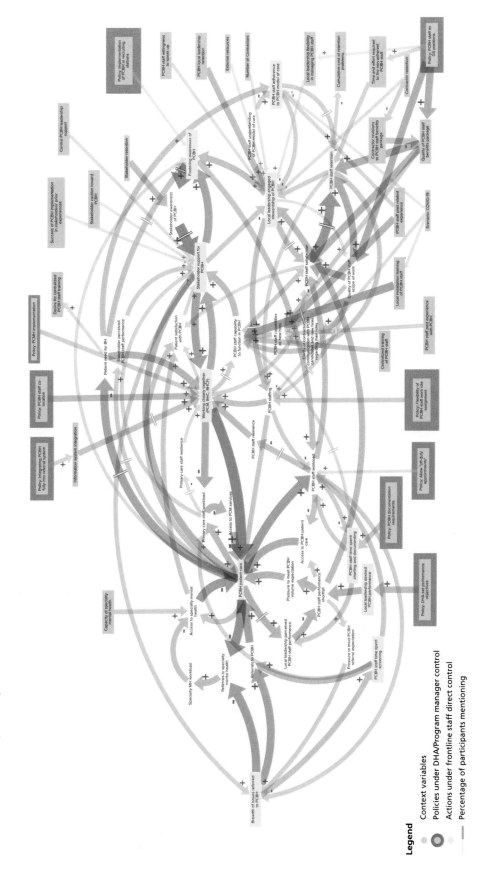

Legend

- Context variables
- Policies under DHA/Program manager control
- Actions under frontline staff direct control
- Percentage of participants mentioning

NOTE: In Kumu, https://RANDCorp.kumu.io/pcbh, this is the *Shared Understanding Diagram–Army* view.

Figure C.3
Shared Understanding—Air Force

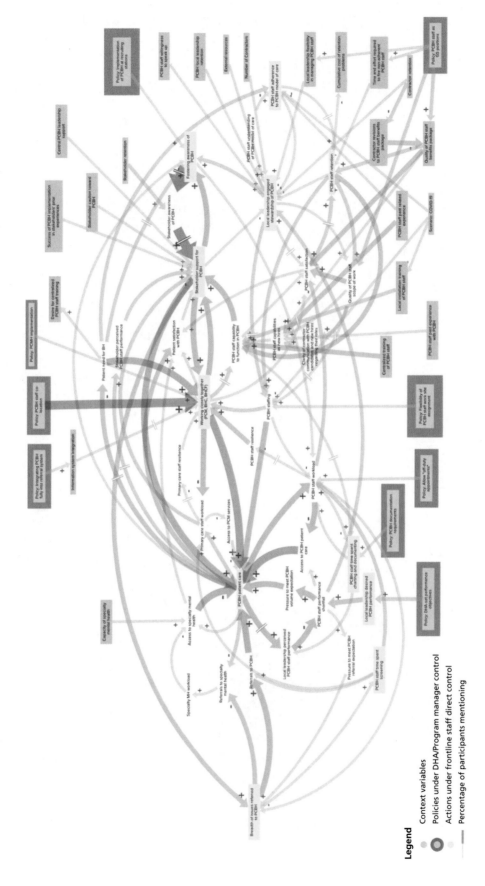

NOTE: In Kumu, https://RANDCorp.kumu.io/pcbh, this is the *Shared Understanding Diagram–Air Force* view.

**Figure C.4
Shared Understanding—Primary Care Managers**

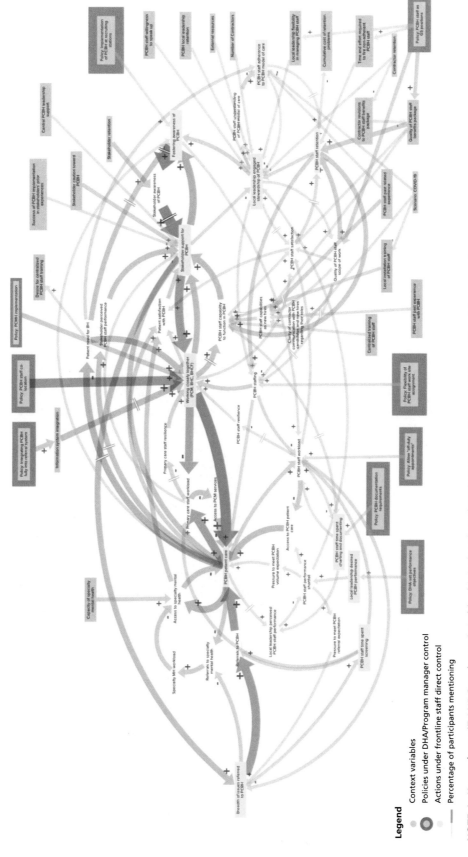

Legend

- Context variables
- Policies under DHA/Program manager control
- Actions under frontline staff direct control
- Percentage of participants mentioning

NOTE: In Kumu, https://RANDCorp.kumu.io/pcbh, this is the *Shared Understanding Diagram—Primary Care Managers* view.

Figure C.5
Shared Understanding—Behavioral Health Care Facilitators

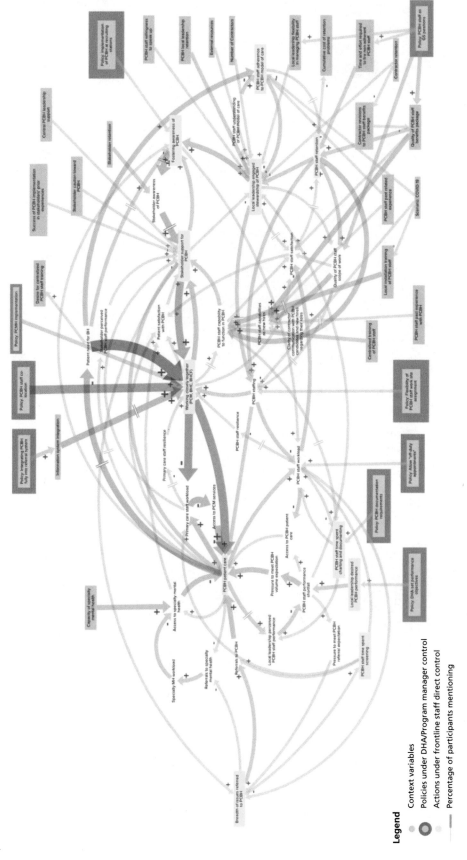

Legend

Context variables
Policies under DHA/Program manager control
Actions under frontline staff direct control
Percentage of participants mentioning

NOTE: In Kumu, https://RANDCorp.kumu.io/pcbh, this is the *Shared Understanding Diagram–Behavioral Health Care Facilitators* view.

Figure C.6
Shared Understanding—Behavioral Health Consultants

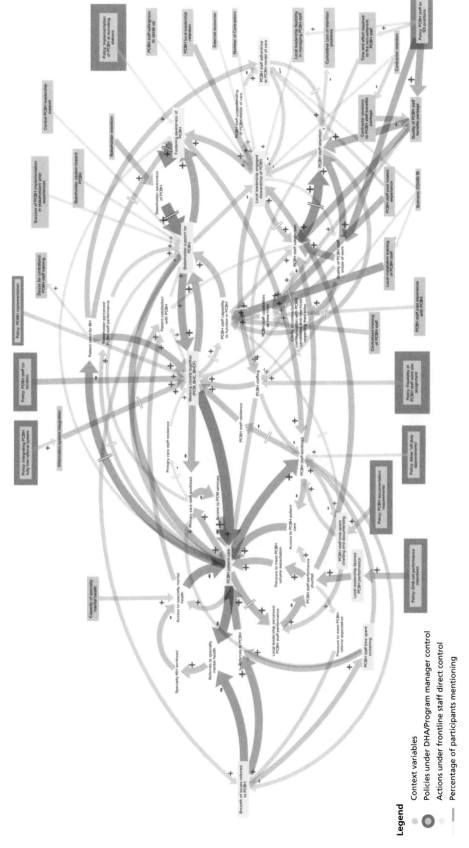

Legend

Context variables

Policies under DHA/Program manager control

Actions under frontline staff direct control

Percentage of participants mentioning

NOTE: In Kumu, https://RANDCorp.kumu.io/pcbh, this is the *Shared Understanding Diagram–Behavioral Health Consultants* view.

Figure C.7
Shared Understanding—Local Leaders

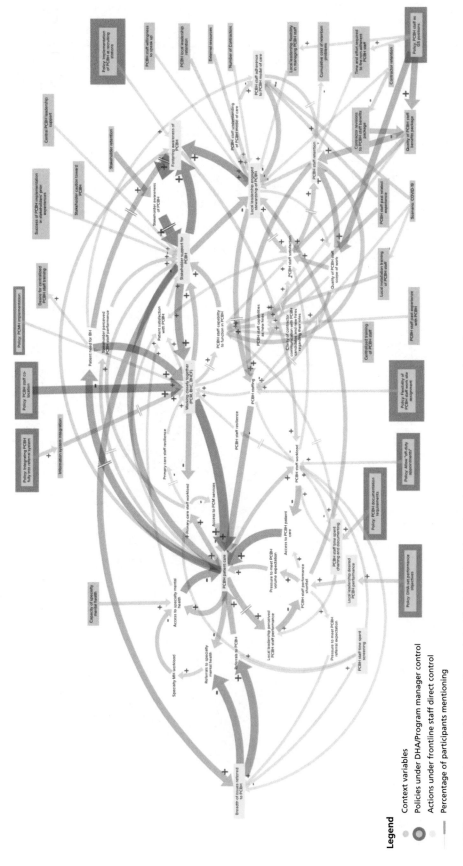

NOTE: In Kumu, https://RANDCorp.kumu.io/pcbh, this is the *Shared Understanding Diagram—Local Leaders* view.

References

Acosta, J. D., A. Becker, J. L. Cerully, M. P. Fisher, L. T. Martin, R. Vardavas, M. E. Slaughter, and T. L. Schell, *Mental Health Stigma in the Military*, Santa Monica, Calif.: RAND Corporation, RR-426-OSD, 2014. As of September 4, 2020:
http://www.rand.org/pubs/research_reports/RR426.html

Colpe, L. J., J. A. Naifeh, P. A. Aliaga, N. A. Sampson, S. G. Heeringa, M. B. Stein, R. J. Ursano, C. S. Fullerton, M. K. Nock, M. L. Schoenbaum, et al., on behalf of the Army STARRS Collaborators, "Mental Health Treatment Among Soldiers with Current Medical Disorders in the Army Study to Assess Risk and Resilience in Service Members," *Military Medicine*, Vol. 180, No. 10, October 2015, pp. 1041–1051. As of February 15, 2021:
https://academic.oup.com/milmed/article/180/10/1041/4160597

Dietrich, A. J., T. E. Oxman, J. W. Williams, Jr., K. Kroenke, C. H. Schulberg, M. Bruce, and S. L. Barry, "Going to Scale: Re-Engineering Systems for Primary Care Treatment of Depression," *Annals of Family Medicine*, Vol. 2, No. 4, August 2014, pp. 301–304.

Eibner, C., J. S. Ringel, B. Kilmer, R. L. Pacula, and C. Diaz, "The Cost of Postdeployment Mental Health and Cognitive Conditions," in T. Tanielian and L. H. Jaycox, eds., *Invisible Wounds of War*, Santa Monica, Calif.: RAND Corporation, MG-720-CCF, 2008, pp. 169–241. As of February 15, 2021:
https://www.rand.org/pubs/monographs/MG720.html

Engel, C. C., "Proposal for a Collaborative Military Primary Care Mental Health Services Quality Improvement Program," *Federal Practitioner*, Vol. 11, No. 11, 1994, pp. 18–29.

Engel, C. C., R. M. Bray, L. H. Jaycox, M. C. Freed, D. Zatzick, M. E. Lane, D. Brambilla, K. R. Olmsted, R. Vandermaas-Peeler, B. Litz, et al., "Implementing Collaborative Primary Care for Depression and Posttraumatic Stress Disorder: Design and Sample for a Randomized Trial in the US Military Health System," *Contemporary Clinical Trials*, Vol. 39, No. 2, 2014, pp. 310–319.

Engel, C. C., L. H. Jaycox, M. C. Freed, R. M. Bray, D. Brambilla, D. F. Zatzick, B. T. Litz, T. Tanielian, L. A. Novak, M. E. Lane, et al., "Centrally Assisted Collaborative Telecare for Posttraumatic Stress Disorder and Depression Among Military Personnel Attending Primary Care: A Randomized Clinical Trial," *JAMA Internal Medicine*, Vol. 176, No. 7, 2016, pp. 948–956. As of February 15, 2021:
https://www.rand.org/pubs/external_publications/EP66510.html

Engel, C. C., K. Kroenke, and W. J. Katon, "Mental Health Services in Army Primary Care: The Need for a Collaborative Health Care Agenda," *Military Medicine*, Vol. 159, No. 3, 1994, pp. 203–209.

Engel, C. C., T. Oxman, C. Yamamoto, D. Gould, S. Barry, P. Stewart, K. Kroenke, J. W. Williams, Jr., and A. J. Dietrich, "RESPECT-MIL: Feasibility of a Systems-level Collaborative Care Approach to Depression and Post-Traumatic Stress Disorder in Military Primary Care," *Military Medicine*, Vol. 173, No. 10, 2008, pp. 935–940. As of February 15, 2021:
https://pubmed.ncbi.nlm.nih.gov/19160608/

Fetters, M. D., L. A. Curry, and J. W. Creswell, "Achieving Integration in Mixed Methods Designs—Principles and Practices," *Health Services Research*, Vol. 48, No. 6, Pt. 2, 2013, pp. 2134–2156.

Fredericks, K. A., M. Deegan, and J. G. Carman, "Using System Dynamics as an Evaluation Tool: Experience from a Demonstration Program," *American Journal of Evaluation*, Vol. 29, No. 3, 2008, pp. 251–267.

Gillock, K. L., C. Zayfert, M. T. Hegel, and R. J. Ferguson, "Posttraumatic Stress Disorder in Primary Care: Prevalence and Relationships with Physical Symptoms and Medical Utilization," *General Hospital Psychiatry*, Vol. 26, No. 6, 2005, pp. 392–399. As of February 15, 2021:
https://www.sciencedirect.com/science/article/pii/S0163834305001118?via%3Dihub

Gureje, O., M. Von Korff, G. E. Simon, and R. Gater, "Persistent Pain and Well-Being: A World Health Organization Study in Primary Care," *Journal of the American Medical Association*, Vol. 280, No. 2, 1998, pp. 147–151. As of February 15, 2021:
https://pubmed.ncbi.nlm.nih.gov/9669787/

Harris, D. M., and J. LeFavour, *Final Evaluation of Navy Medicine's Behavioral Health Integration Program (BHIP) Two-Year Demonstration Project*, Alexandria, Va.: Center for Naval Analyses, 2005.

Harris, D. M., and S. D. Tela, *Organization for Optimization: Intervention Recommendations for Optimizing the Delivery of Ambulatory Primary Care and Mental Health Care in Navy Military Treatment Facilities*, Alexandria, Va.: Center for Naval Analyses, 2002.

Hoge, C. W., J. L. Auchterlonie, and C. S. Milliken, "Mental Health Problems, Use of Mental Health Services, and Attrition from Military Service After Returning from Deployment to Iraq or Afghanistan," *Journal of the American Medical Association*, Vol. 295, No. 9, 2006, pp. 1023–1032.

Hoge, C. W., S. H. Grossman, J. L. Auchterlonie, L. A. Riviere, C. S. Milliken, and J. E. Wilk, "PTSD Treatment for Soldiers After Combat Deployment: Low Utilization of Mental Health Care and Reasons for Dropout," *Psychiatric Services*, Vol. 65, No. 8, 2014, pp. 997–1004.

Hoge, C. W., S. E. Lesikar, and R. Guevara, "Mental Disorders Among US Military Personnel in the 1990s: Association with High Levels of Healthcare Utilization and Early Military Attrition," *American Journal of Psychiatry*, Vol. 159, No. 9, 2002, pp. 1576–1583.

Hoge, C. W., A. Terhakopian, C. A. Castro, S. C. Messer, and C. C. Engel, "Association of Posttraumatic Stress Disorder with Somatic Symptoms, Healthcare Visits, and Absenteeism Among Iraq War Veterans," *American Journal of Psychiatry*, Vol. 164, No. 1, 2007, pp. 150–153.

Hunter, C. L., J. L. Goodie, A. C. Dobmeyer, and K. A. Dorrance, "Tipping Points in the Department of Defense's Experience with Psychologists in Primary Care," *American Psychologist*, Vol. 69, No. 4, 2014, pp. 388–398. As of February 15, 2021:
https://psycnet.apa.org/record/2014-16756-007?doi=1

Ivankova, N. V., J. W. Creswell, and S. Stick, "Using Mixed-Methods Sequential Explanatory Design: From Theory to Practice," *Field Methods*, Vol. 18, No. 1, 2006, pp. 3–20.

Jaén, C., and R. Palmer, "Shorter Adaptive Reserve Measures," *Annals of Family Medicine*, Vol. 8 (Suppl. 1), 2012, pp. 1–2.

Kessler, R. C., P. de Jonge, V. Shahly, H. M. van Loo, P. S.-E. Wang, and M. A. Wilcox, "Epidemiology of Depression," in I. H. Gotlib and C. L. Hammen, eds., *Handbook of Depression*, New York: Guilford Press, 2014, pp. 7–24.

Kroenke, K., R. L. Spitzer, J. B. W. Williams, P. O. Monahan, and B. Lowe, "Anxiety Disorders in Primary Care: Prevalence, Impairment, Comorbidity, and Detection," *Annals of Internal Medicine*, Vol. 146, No. 5, March 2007, pp. 317–325. As of February 15, 2021:
https://pubmed.ncbi.nlm.nih.gov/17339617/

Lazar, S. G., "The Mental Health Needs of Military Service Members and Veterans," *Psychodynamic Psychiatry*, Vol. 42, No. 3, 2014, pp. 459–478. As of Febrauary 15, 2021:
https://guilfordjournals.com/doi/10.1521/pdps.2014.42.3.459

Liebschutz, J., R. Saitz, V. Brower, T. M. Keane, C. Lloyd-Travaglini, T. Averbuch, and J. H. Samet, "PTSD in Urban Primary Care: High Prevalence and Low Physician Recognition," *Society of General Internal Medicine*, Vol. 22, No. 6, June 2007, pp. 719–726.

Meadows, S. O., C. C. Engel, R. L. Collins, R. L. Beckman, J. Breslau, E. L. Bloom, M. S. Dunbar, M. L. Gilbert, D. M. Grant, J. Hawes-Dawson, S. B. Holliday, S. MacCarthy, E. R. Pedersen, M. Robbins, A. J. Rose, J. Ryan, T. L. Schell, and M. Simmons, *2018 Department of Defense Health Related Behaviors Survey (HRBS): Results for the Active Component*, Santa Monica, Calif.: RAND Corporation, RR-4222-OSD, 2021. As of June 23, 2021:
https://www.rand.org/pubs/research_reports/RR4222.html

Meadows, S. O., C. C. Engel, R. L. Collins, R. L. Beckman, M. Cefalu, J. Hawes-Dawson, M. Waymouth, A. M. Kress, L. Sontag-Padilla, R. Ramchand, and K. M. Williams, *2015 Department of Defense Health Related Behaviors Survey (HRBS)*, Santa Monica, Calif.: RAND Corporation, RR-1695-OSD, 2018. As of September 4, 2020:
https://www.rand.org/pubs/research_reports/RR1695.html

Meadows, S. O., L. L. Miller, and S. Robson, *Airman and Family Resilience: Lessons from the Scientific Literature*, Santa Monica, Calif.: RAND Corporation, RR-106-AF, 2015. As of February 15, 2021:
http://www.rand.org/pubs/research_reports/RR106.html

Miller, W. L., B. F. Crabtree, P. A. Nutting, K. C. Stange, and C. R. Jaén, "Primary Care Practice Development: A Relationship-Centered Approach," *Annals of Family Medicine*, Vol. 8 (Suppl. 1), 2010, pp. S68–S79.

Nutting, P. A., W. L. Miller, B. F. Crabtree, C. R. Jaén, E. E. Stewart, and K. C. Stange, "Initial Lessons from the First National Demonstration Project on Practice Transformation to a Patient-Centered Medical Home," *Annals of Family Medicine*, Vol. 7, No. 3, 2009, pp. 254–260.

Oxman, T. E., A. J. Dietrich, J. W. Williams, Jr., and K. Kroenke, "A Three-Component Model for Engineering Systems for the Treatment of Depression in Primary Care," *Psychosomatics*, Vol. 43, No. 6, 2002, pp. 441–450.

Rosellini, A. J., S. G. Heeringa, M. B. Stein, R. J. Ursano, W. T. Chiu, L. J. Colpe, C. S. Fullerton, S. E. Gilman, I. Hwang, J. A. Naifeh, et al., "Lifetime Prevalence of DSM-IV Mental Disorders Among New Soldiers in the U.S. Army: Results from the Army Study to Assess Risk and Resilience in Service Members (ARMY STARRS)," *Depression and Anxiety*, Vol. 32, 2015, pp. 13–24.

Runyan, C., V. P. Fonseca, J. G. Meyer, M. S. Oordt, and G. W. Talcott, "A Novel Approach for Mental Health Disease Management: The Air Force Medical Service's Interdisciplinary Model," *Disease Management*, Vol. 6, 2003, pp. 179–187.

Rush, T., C. A. LeardMann, and N. F. Crum-Cianflone, "Obesity and Associated Adverse Health Outcomes Among U.S. Military Members and Veterans: Findings from the Millennium Cohort Study," *Obesity*, Vol. 24, No. 7, 2016, pp. 1582–1589.

Sharp, M. L., N. T. Fear, R. J. Rona, S. Wessely, N. Greenberg, N. Jones, and L. Goodwin, "Stigma as a Barrier to Seeking Health Care Among Military Personnel with Mental Health Problems," *Epidemiologic Review*, Vol. 37, January 2015, pp. 144–162.

Stahlman, S., and A. A. Oetting, "Mental Health Disorders and Mental Health Problems, Active Component, U.S. Armed Forces, 2007–2016," *Medical Surveillance Monthly Report*, Vol. 25, No. 3, 2018, pp. 2–11.

Sterman, J. D., *Business Dynamics: Systems Thinking and Modeling for a Complex World*, Boston: Irwin/McGraw-Hill, 2000.

Tanielian, T. L., and L. H. Jaycox, *Invisible Wounds of War: Psychological and Cognitive Injuries, Their Consequences, and Services to Assist Recovery*, Santa Monica, Calif.: RAND Corporation, MG-720-CCF, 2008. As of September 4, 2020:
https://www.rand.org/pubs/monographs/MG720.html

Toblin, R. L., P. J. Quartana, L. A. Riviere, K. C. Walper, and C. W. Hoge, "Chronic Pain and Opioid Use in U.S. Soldiers After Combat Deployment," *JAMA Internal Medicine*, Vol. 174, No. 8, 2014, pp. 1400–1401.

Tomoaia-Cotisel, A., "The Journey Toward the Patient-Centered Medical Home: A Grounded Dynamic Theory of Primary Care Transformation," thesis, London School of Hygiene and Tropical Medicine, 2018. As of February 15, 2021:
https://researchonline.lshtm.ac.uk/id/eprint/4647856/

Troxel, W. M., R. A. Shih, E. R. Pedersen, L. Geyer, M. P. Fisher, B. A. Griffin, A. C. Haas, J. R. Kurz, and P. S. Steinberg, *Sleep in the Military: Promoting Healthy Sleep Among U.S. Servicemembers*, Santa Monica, Calif.: RAND Corporation, RR-739-OSD, 2015. As of September 4, 2020:
http://www.rand.org/pubs/research_reports/RR739.html

Wong, E. C., L. H. Jaycox, and L. A. Ayer, *Evaluating the Implementation of Re-Engineering Systems of Primary Care Treatment in the Military (RESPECT-MIL)*, Santa Monica, Calif.: RAND Corporation, RR-588-OSD, 2015. As of September 4, 2020:
https://www.rand.org/pubs/research_reports/RR588.html